Praise

'Dan Moore is one of the top fitness coaches in the UK. A true professional and expert in the industry. This book isn't just about fitness, it's about self-improvement overall. If you're looking to maximise your potential, read Dan's book.'
—**Paul Mort**, bestselling author and 2 x master coach of the Year

'Dan is the leader in his field, having changed hundreds of people's lives for the better, both physically and mentally. If you're reading this book then you're in good hands, as Dan's passion for what he does is infectious. I hope he inspires you like he has myself and many others.'
—**Ben Davis**, Founder Fitness Marketing Agency

'In my travels around the world speaking about the business of fitness, I have met a LOT of gym owners and can say with some credibility, Dan is the cream of the crop. Dan's ability to balance confident action-taking with a humility and unquenchable hunger to learn is a dynamite combo.'
—**Mark Fisher**, Speaker, coach and founder of Mark Fisher Fitness

D1407507

The blueprint and
mindset you
need to live a
healthy life

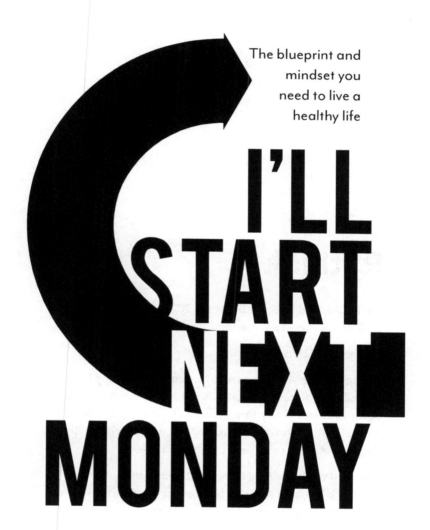

I'LL START NEXT MONDAY

DAN MOORE

R^ethink

First published in Great Britain in 2022
by Rethink Press (www.rethinkpress.com)

© Copyright Dan Moore

*To Aimee, for pushing me to do this book
when it was only an idea*

*To Mum and Dad, for getting me into books from an
early age – I have learned a lot from reading*

*And to Beau and Macy – I hope you enjoy reading
this when you are older*

Contents

Introduction

'**I**'ll start next Monday.'

How many times have you said that to yourself? Great intentions, fresh ideas, New Year's resolutions … You know *what* to do, but you just can't quite seem to get into it or sustain it.

I find it fascinating that the world is getting sicker, the fitness industry has skyrocketed over the past ten years and there's more information out there than ever before, and yet people are still stuck. You may have 'failed' in the past – with gyms, trainers or the latest diet. The chances are you are probably great at other things in life such as parenting, being a good husband or wife and making progress with your business or career, but your health is the one thing you can't quite nail down. It's not only about knowing *what* to do but also about having the selfishness to look after number one.

I would have you consider that looking after *you* is the most selfless thing you could do. Without striving to be the best version of you – physically, mentally, in your energy and confidence – then how can you expect to be consistently productive? Yes, your kids are your life and your career is hugely important – I get that, and I feel the same. But there comes a point where you need to realise how much value you would be adding to the people close to you by being happy and confident, knowing you're protecting your own energy and confidence.

The fact of the matter is, your mindset will ensure you do not 'give up' as a parent or with your career, so why do you accept that your physical and mental wellbeing are less important, or that becoming healthier just isn't meant to be? You know deep down that anything good you have achieved in life has come through overcoming obstacles and working through stress rather than avoiding challenges or relying solely on willpower or motivation.

You cannot build a better career or business with a limiting mindset, and the same goes for your own health. You cannot improve your long-term fitness with certain beliefs or habits, and I want to help you change those.

No more not doing what you said you would. In this book I want to help you change your mindset and lifestyle. I want to help you find out what works for you.

I have been in the health and fitness industry for ten years now, from working in parks as a personal trainer to now running a gym, with staff and around 250 clients. It has been a fun ride, even though there have of course been stresses. That's not only the day-to-day business stress, together with the usual excitement, highs and lows, but also having to balance all that with being a husband and dad to two girls, while also looking after my own health and fitness.

The much sought-after balance is tough to nail down. Having a business in the health and fitness industry, and having previously been a professional footballer, I get that it's hard. And this is my life, where health and fitness are what I am passionate about. For you, it's likely even harder. The idea of living a life where your body is an asset, where you have more energy, you feel confident within, and you're the role model you want to be, probably makes complete sense to you. You know you need to do it and you know it's good for you, but there always seems to be a good reason why something else is more important.

I hope this book can help with that.

I feel personal training and gyms in general are the solution, but you have probably had your fingers burnt in the past. Maybe you just haven't yet found what works for you. You start, you stop, the cycle continues, and it gets tougher and tougher every time you try and kickstart yourself back into action.

Don't get me wrong – I am not going to say I know what it's like to be out of shape and that I hate fitness, because that just isn't me. I haven't built my business through my own personal struggle with fitness. Before I became a trainer, I was a professional athlete, but I do know the principles of growing a business, employing staff and having a young family, as I do, are remarkably similar.

When I started out, I may have been in shape physically, but I did not really know where my life was going. My now wife Aimee and I had been together for a year, and we didn't really know what path we were on or what we wanted to do in the longer term. We had no money, no real qualifications and no unique skillsets for the careers we wanted to have. Something had to change.

Our own get-up-and-go, the help of mentors in specific areas and a huge mindset shift over the last ten years, together with other things I've written about in this book, have helped us build a business we love. We have also helped hundreds of current and past clients change their lifestyle habits by adopting a different approach. We haven't only created an approach – we've created a movement that now continues to move without us. We have created a community bigger than ourselves. People love coming to our gym, and I am proud of that.

Here's something that might sound odd: I don't like gyms either.

That's why we created a gym for other people who don't like gyms.

There's no doubt that's what people need – to be part of something they enjoy.

Our vision was to create a safe, non-judgemental space for busy professionals who struggle to find time for something they want to do and can enjoy. This is all built on the foundation of beliefs that I use, apply to my own life and strongly attribute to the growth of our business and community.

We have gone from 30 members to now around 250 and have since moved to a bigger location. I have travelled the world, visiting the best gyms from London to New York. I have joined fitness retreats from Loch Ness to Bali, and I have worked with some incredible mentors in our industry. I love pushing myself out of my own comfort zone while learning and striving to make everything better. Even writing this book has been a challenge and something I'd never have imagined myself doing. You have to get comfortable with the unknown, though, so I decided to write about everything I have learned and taught over the last ten years in the fitness industry.

In those ten years, the biggest lesson for me and for my clients has been that there's no point absorbing more and more information unless you're willing to act on what you are learning. I want you to learn something and apply it to your own life. Even if that is only one small mindset shift or a new belief, or if you learn to slow down and think so that you can speed back up again, for me this book would have achieved its aims. I want you to get inspired and to think differently about yourself and your journey. To understand what it takes to change and learn how to enjoy the process. Imagine that.

By the end of this book, I hope you will be inspired to act on some of the things I have learned over the last ten years, in how to improve your fitness, wellbeing and mindset, and in how to make long-term changes to your lifestyle. By making those changes, you will probably also inspire your friends and family. You can do all this, but it starts with you. Be the catalyst and the driving force for you, your family, your kids' future, your career … whatever inspires you the most.

Your health is your number one asset in anything you want to do with your life.

Let's get to it.

This book is a blueprint for how I live my life and for how I have helped change the lives of the people who have been part of our gym since we founded it.

Read this book, take action and enjoy improving your life.

You might have been wondering what the title of this book is about. It's likely that until now you have taken the 'I'll start next Monday' approach. I'm sure you've already found that it's easy to skip a Monday – of fitness and of focusing on you – because you've had a heavy weekend or you have too much work on. That sets the tone for the rest of your week, then you promise yourself you'll start *next* Monday, even though you deep down know you won't. The more often you do this, the more it stresses you out, and the less likely it becomes that you'll get stuff done. After reading this, you'll be able to change to the 'Never miss a Monday' mindset, which you can take forward with you for the rest of your life. One day you will thank me for it, both physically and mentally.

Never miss a Monday.

If you have any questions after reading this book, or if you ever want to reach out and chat about your own health, fitness or mindset, email me at dan@dmelite.co.uk.

PART ONE
MINDSET

When people think about bettering themselves, they are often tempted to focus on the programme, the features or benefits, and on what they need to do to get from A to B. For example, if you want to lose weight, you know you need to eat less food and start moving more – and more efficiently – by walking and going to the gym. We all know that works. Often, though, we do not seem to be able to do it, even though we *know* it's what we want and that it will make our lives better. We still fall into the trap of either not doing it at all or not sticking at it.

That is not a skillset issue or a process issue. It is a mindset issue.

You don't need more information – you need more action. Confidence and progression come through *doing*.

When you don't understand the underlying reasons for why you are doing something and why it is important, the chances are you will revert back to what you know and feel comfortable with. How many times have you been in a good routine, then something throws you, you stop the routine and you never get back into it?

To see goals through and move to the next level, you need to move your mindset to the next level. If you don't bring your mindset along for the ride, it will always pull you back. That's why it is important you confront your mindset *before* you consider how you should train, what you should eat, which supplements you should take – all the questions that will arise when you start out on your fitness journey.

In this part of the book, we will look at the three key elements of mindset:

1. Confidence

2. Character

3. Clarity

These are deep topics, and I want to get you thinking differently about all of them. That's because to become different – to get to a different place – you need to think differently. Remember: what got you where you are now won't get you to the new place you want to be.

ONE

Confidence

Have you ever played on a computer game and looked for a cheat code? When you get the code, your mind is blown as you easily move to another level. That's how I see confidence – as soon as your confidence improves, it has an immediate, positive effect on just about everything else in your life.

If you lack confidence, you are always limited in some way. Here's the good news: like all the topics in this book, confidence is a skill that can be worked at. There is no doubt that some people are born with natural confidence, but a lot of the confident people you know have had to work hard to get there. People who lack confidence are likely to claim 'That's just not me' or 'I have never been confident and I never will be'. They simply accept their situation, believing they can never feel differently.

My confidence has grown a huge amount, because I have worked at it. When I was younger, I was always shy and introverted. Over the years, pushing myself out of my comfort zones in different areas has increased my confidence. My increased confidence makes it easier now to try new things without worrying as much about failing. I don't think anyone who met me now would think I had ever struggled with confidence. However confident you become, though, there are still times you are tested and must stand up to it.

When I was about eighteen years old, I played football with professionals who were senior to me. They all looked naturally confident, and when I watched myself back, it was terrible. I was incredibly nervous watching the playback, and if there had been a trapdoor in the room, I would have opened it and disappeared.

Ten years on, I was creating my own videos for members of our gym and couldn't believe how my confidence had grown. It doesn't happen overnight, but when you find your confidence has grown, it's amazing to see how that changes your whole attitude to life.

I still have room to grow. I am sure you do too, which is why you are reading this book. So let's work at it.

Have you got skin in the game?

How many times have you got free stuff you haven't really valued? You can now watch endless content free on YouTube, but do you remember much of it? There are free workouts on YouTube, but it's unlikely you will follow them religiously four times per week.

The same goes for content on health and fitness. There is more free information and content available now than ever before, and the fitness industry is exploding, yet there are more obese people in the western world than ever before. So why is that? It certainly isn't an information problem. It's an *implementation* issue.

I do not mean that paying money is enough in itself, but it does mean you are much more likely to be invested in what you are doing.

I believe this book will change your mindset if you read it, reread it and take notes on what you have learned. If my advice leads to one significant change in your lifestyle, that's a huge success to me, and I know it can be the catalyst for more. All that comes through you investing in yourself by buying this book.

I have had mentors in the past I could not really afford, and I would not advise you get yourself into debt to help you move forward. I remember being so desperate to go to events and learn from successful people that I would max out credit cards to know that stuff. You could argue, though, that credit cards and debt are good for investing in appreciating assets. And there are no bigger appreciating assets than you, your health and how you think.

I realise I am speaking here more from a personal development perspective than about fitness and the gym, but the same principles apply. You may well have had memberships at gyms with excellent equipment, but did you get anything out of that? How many times did you go over the two or three years you were a member? If you paid more for membership at a gym that fully supported you in committing your time and energy, wouldn't you get better results?

And please do not be fooled by the pay-as-you-go (PAYG) trap, which leaves the motivation up to you. It's likely that you will not be motivated 99% of the time, which is doing you no favours. PAYG only tempts you *not* to do it. If you're tired on Monday morning and you have a PAYG session at the gym, you probably won't show up. This also affects the quality of the gym – if we had only PAYG members, we would not be able to have such a strong business, create the community we have or help change so many lives in the way we do.

If you buy cheap, you buy twice. How often have you bought a cheaper solution, only to buy the same standard of product two or three times over? The two or three products don't do the job as well and don't last as long as if you had bought a higher-quality product in the first place.

If you feel your gym is too expensive, think about how you will feel ten years later when you need surgery for back pain, for example. Or think about how you will feel after gaining weight over the next few years, meaning you can't wear the clothes you want to wear or do things you want to do.

What is the price you pay for the above in time, mental energy, stress, what you cannot do and maybe money? I know if I didn't invest, I would not have a gym now. I would go as far as to say I wouldn't be in the fitness industry. If I did not pay the price I would not have the business I love that serves other people and I would be in a job I did not like.

I definitely paid the price for the first few years both with the amount I worked, giving up weekends as I had football on Saturdays, so I would work most Sundays. Rather than weekly nights out, I invested in coaches that could propel me forward and help me understand what to do and how to future plan me and my business. Truth is when you work for yourself on your own, it's a job you have created for yourself without paid holidays and a pension. As much as I enjoyed it at the time, I knew further down the line it would be hard to maintain, so I sought out coaching.

Getting started

Every time I work with a new client, I emphasise the importance of just getting started.

Sometimes we can look too far ahead, overthink our longer-term goals and want results yesterday. We are all guilty of that to some extent, but we also know deep down that all good things take time. You simply can't instantly get to where you want to be, whether that's on your fitness journey, in your career, when you start a new business or when you first become a parent. I remember being scared witless when we went home with our first newborn, feeling completely unsure about what we needed to do, and it took time to adopt all the new habits I needed to feel confident in looking after Beau.

You don't ever become great at something overnight. Success takes time, and long before you get remotely close to where you want to go, you need to get started. It is nearly always tough at the beginning to start on a new fitness and lifestyle journey – the thought of stepping into a new environment, cutting back on the food and drink you're used to, or experiencing the soreness that comes from new exercise. But as long as you ride that out, you will soon find a new comfort zone.

You could always say 'I'll start next Monday' or look for reasons *not* to make a start. But you won't keep buying that, and over time it will tire you out making excuses to yourself.

Step one is exactly that. Get started one way or another. Do not overthink what you need to do, and simply aim to take imperfect action.

When we started our gym business or moved location, if we had overthought the situation, we would not have done anything. If we hadn't done anything, we would not have created the community we have now, together with the staff we are so lucky to work with. When we opened the gym at our first location, we had no money and no plan – we simply opened it because it seemed a cool idea to have our own place. At the start we only had a few clients and a vision of making our and their lives better. We weren't a company as such back then, so all the risk was personal. We had just moved house, and I had no real clue about how to run a gym, so it was a stressful time. Staff management, Facebook ads and business plans were not even in my mind. Our accounts were all over the place, and I only ever thought one month ahead at a time.

Would I ever have set up the gym if I'd known what was involved? Probably not. If I'd overthought it at the time, would we be where we are now? Definitely not. Now I'm incredibly relieved that we took the plunge without overthinking everything. Success is all about balance and making sure you trust your own judgement, but sometimes you need to be ready to take a risk in getting started.

I am not saying it's always wise to go blindly into things without knowing the worst-case scenario and with a 'build it and they will come' mentality. But I have learnt that sometimes you must make that call and move forward with whatever you want to get started on.

I also know that with many new ideas, which for you likely includes the idea of joining a gym to get fit, we overthink the mechanics as an excuse or reason to slow us down and stay where we are. It might well be that you have previously had negative experiences in a gym environment or of working with a personal trainer. I get that – we hear it a lot from our clients. However, don't use that as an excuse or let it put you off giving yourself another chance.

There is something out there that works for you, which you will enjoy. In the meantime, there are lots of things you can do to get started on your own.

One of the best ways to start is by creating simple boundaries. Here are some examples:

- Being more disciplined in your sleep routine

- Completing a walk each day and getting used to a daily step count

- Embracing an awareness of your food choices so you can immediately reduce calories without a huge amount of thought

- Trying some at-home workouts

If you feel you need some extra help from an expert, reach out. If I hadn't sought business help, I certainly wouldn't be running a gym now. I may not even have become a personal trainer if I hadn't asked for help from people who had done the same and who helped me to eliminate mistakes. It's not always easy sending that first message or making that first call, but having peer support from other people – fellow gym goers, walking buddies or a personal trainer – and using the help wisely will take you to your next level of fitness.

In his book *Atomic Habits*, James Clear explains how to make tiny changes and achieve remarkable results. Here's a quote that I find inspiring:

'Where to focus: For the beginner, execution. For the intermediate, strategy. For the expert, mindset.'

You will develop better habits, becoming more educated and more of an expert over time. Remember, though, that *everyone* starts out as a beginner, getting started and doing the work. That said, mindset is as essential in the beginning as it is in retaining your new position.

CASE STUDY: CALUM RICHARDSON

Calum signed up with us because he didn't feel good and wanted to lose some weight. He says that soon after he started, he realised that there was no quick fix, and that he needed to develop his mindset in order to achieve and maintain weight loss. He realised how small changes in his lifestyle could lead to big changes in his life. He also learned he was benefiting from more than only losing weight.

By week 50, Calum had lost 2 stone and found he was able to change his main focus to maintaining his new lifestyle and toning up. He feels certain that his improved wellbeing enabled him to enjoy his best year in business in thirteen years. He also says his new mindset has made him feel calmer and better able to enjoy time with his children and family.

Calum feels that setting himself clear weekly goals has led to an increase in his confidence, energy, focus and productivity levels.

Upper limits vs lower limits

Before you start, you need to gauge what you can realistically set out to achieve. There is no point saying you want to lose four stone over the next few months if you won't be able to commit the time or energy to the process. You *can* still get there in the end, but it is likely to take you longer. You also may not be able to train five times per week and give up all your favourite foods in the same way someone else you know has done it.

Remember that your goals must align with what you're able *and willing* to commit to.

Key here is recognising your upper limit and your lower limit. Your upper limit is your ideal – what you can aim to achieve on a day when you have more time and energy. Your lower limit is the minimum – what you can easily stick to for 90% of the time.

Look at the three 'big rocks' in your lifestyle – your steps/movement, diet/hydration and sleep – and commit to doing what you can stick to on upper- and lower-limit days.

Here are some examples:

Steps/movement

When you are at the gym or doing a home workout for 45 minutes, you know you are compounding the calorie burn and movement with your steps (upper limit).

On a day where you are tighter for time and not doing a structured workout, you may get in 7–10,000 steps (lower limit).

Diet/hydration

Your ideal plan may be achieving a calorie deficit, with only 1,500 calories per day (upper limit).

Then some days you can't be as bothered tracking calories and you have a meal out, so you end up closer to 2,000 calories (lower limit).

If you aren't into tracking calories, you may just know that an upper-limit day would be three meals without any snacking, with three litres of water. On a lower-limit day, you might have a couple of snacks during the day, a takeaway in the evening and slightly less water.

Sleep

In an ideal scenario, you might be able to get eight or nine hours' sleep per night (upper limit).

Within your control – if you can sleep well and aren't disturbed by your kids – you know that if you go to bed on time, you can get a minimum of seven hours' sleep per night (lower limit).

Every time you make it to the gym and/or have a solid day diet-wise, it buys you a rest day or down time to enjoy what you want without stressing about it.

One of the biggest mistakes people make is repeatedly starting and stopping their fitness plans completely. Once you recognise your upper and lower limits, if you have a day where you're extra busy at work, your kids have a lot on or you're stressed and tight for time, you can still stay on track. This is all about doing something, keeping good habits up and maintaining momentum.

Based on the examples above: if you get seven hours of sleep, you're aware of your water intake, you do something movement-based (even if it's just a walk) and have a snack or two in addition to your three meals, it may not be perfect, but it's still fine and you won't feel you've failed. It could still be huge progress from where you started, and over time, the by-product of this thinking will be the results. Small hinges swing big doors. Do you think you would make progress even if you completed 365 lower-limit days? I think so.

Your fitness journey does not have to be perfect. It doesn't have to be all or nothing. It doesn't have to rely on you always having time, and your life doesn't need to be free of stress, because that is impossible. It also doesn't rely on a huge amount of planning. How many times previously have you started a new fitness programme, done too much too soon and then got bored, burnt out or maybe even injured?

Small daily habits – if done consistently – *will* compound over time. Then, when your confidence builds, time allows and your body gets used to the process, it's likely you'll find yourself having more upper-limit days. For me, having a gym and being a personal trainer, running my own business, managing staff and having kids at home, I know how hard it can be to make time to look after yourself. You're not always going to be able to achieve what that person at work says they do or what your friend manages to fit into their schedule. Some days you have to be content with doing the bare minimum.

My task for you after reading this is to start considering the following two questions, depending on where you are now on your journey:

1. What do your upper-limit days look like?

2. What do your lower-limit days look like?

At the end of this chapter, you will find a task on how to record your personal plan of upper limits and lower limits.

Anticipating obstacles

'Plans don't always work, but planning does.'

This statement, made by a mentor of mine, Mark Fisher, holds a lot of truth. You cannot plan everything perfectly, avoiding anything going wrong, but you can have an *ideal* plan – a default – similar to the upper limit discussed in the previous section.

We can be too reactive to situations and blame the situation we're in, as if it has never happened to us before, when it probably has. For example, when Monday morning arrives, it can feel like we have been hit by a train, and we find ourselves reacting negatively to all the challenges of the new week. Could you be more proactive going into Monday rather than letting it happen to you? For example, if you know the start of the week will be tough, you could clear a load of emails on Sunday evening, make sure you get a good night's sleep, and resolve to have a positive mindset on Monday.

If you anticipate obstacles,
you can plan ahead and find
ways to avoid them.

After reading this section of the book, I want you to go away and think more proactively about your fitness and wellbeing and what you can do to stop making the same mistakes over and over. For example, saying you're too busy is not always a valid excuse. Most of the time you'll be able to find someone with more to do who is making more progress than you. That means this is not a busyness issue – it's a planning and implementation issue.

When you find ways to make time for what you want to do, you will get more done and feel a lot better about what you are achieving. You also won't lose time for other stuff, so you'll still be able to achieve higher-value tasks.

Another example of anticipating obstacles is when you do warmups, cool-downs or mobility work to avoid injury. You are being proactive with pain and injury.

A lot of people start out well on their fitness journey but then something stops them, and it may well be the same thing that has stopped them previously. Here are some examples, each with a way to anticipate and/or avoid the obstacle:

- **Injury, from doing too much too soon**

  Make sure you pace yourself correctly, if possible with help from a personal trainer.

- **Hitting an event or time in the year where it's suddenly hard to see the point in continuing**

  You've probably hit this point in previous years, so prepare your mindset in advance and/or decide to take some time out over that point in the year.

- **Being too restrictive with food and ending up bored**

  Think of your upper and lower limits, making sure you allow yourself to have days that aren't as restrictive.

- **Pushing past goals, becoming content with the results then gradually slowing down**

  Accept, for example, that you can't lose weight forever, but you can keep building your strength and use fitness to improve your life.

- **Experiencing a mental block – becoming complacent or looking for a reason to stop after reaching a certain stage**

  This sounds strange but it does happen – you tell yourself you don't deserve to feel good, that this 'isn't you' and that you should revert to what you know. Now this does take some deeper work, but it is worth being aware that the devil voice on your shoulder exists.

Your actions are a good indicator of what you prioritise. You know you should go for that run. Attend that session you booked in. Eat what you planned to rather than having something more convenient. Stick with working with your coach for accountability, as you know you can only do so much on your own.

I have experienced limiting beliefs lots of times over my life. For example, when I played football, I could have pushed harder and been mentally tougher, but I took the easier option and blamed my manager. In fact, I wasn't applying myself correctly, so my limitations were all on me.

I am lucky to have a clearer perspective on this now, but I admit I still have some limiting beliefs in terms of how far we can grow the business. Members of my family haven't run their own businesses, so I find it easier not to take risks (and of course it is sometimes very sensible not to). Every time we consider steps to grow the business, I can hear the worry in my dad's voice, which makes me want to slow down and protect what we have, but sometimes you *must* push and grow.

Limiting beliefs are a real obstacle. The first thing you need to do is to be aware of those beliefs and work at overcoming them. Like anything else, awareness precedes change.

When it comes to your fitness journey, you maybe feel 'it's just not me' – that you're not meant to be fit and healthy because you have never considered yourself to be. Maybe after a busy weekend or a holiday, or if you've had a bad day or week, you cannot psyche yourself up to get back into fitness, so you let things slide. Maybe feeling stressed, or a lack of time leads to limiting beliefs, where looking after yourself is the first thing that goes out of the window.

Whatever usually happens does not have to keep slowing you down or making you stop. It's easy to stop, and it's harder to win and win consistently, but overcoming obstacles will make you feel even better about yourself. Things out of your control will always happen to you, but you can decide how you react to those things. For example, if you have your own business, you will face unexpected challenges every day. Do you deal with each challenge or shun it off? If you shun it off, that challenge will come at you ten times harder down the line, and you probably won't be in business for long. Like anything in life, if you aren't willing to pay the price now – in money, time and effort – you will pay the price down the line.

The super-powerful thing here is that you always have a choice on how to approach each obstacle.

I set aside an hour most days to deal with things that are not in the diary. Certain days and times of the year will generate more challenges, and it helps to be aware of that. I always try and have three to six months of living expenses set aside in case something unexpected happens. If it never happens, then great, but at least you know you can deal with it if it does. I prefer to have some emergency funds rather than spending money for the sake of it – it means I can sleep easier and feel less stressed about things potentially going wrong.

The best thing about anticipating obstacles – just as with upper and lower limits – is that simply being aware of them brings the biggest results. And when you get better at addressing and growing past goals, limiting beliefs and other variables outside of your control, you know you'll be able to do it next time, which builds confidence and resilience.

CASE STUDY: LORIEN CAMERON-ROSS

Since Lorien joined our gym nearly five years ago, she has enjoyed the physical benefits of losing weight and getting fitter and stronger, which she says never gets boring.

Lorien had very clear obstacles to overcome before reaching this point. In December 2018 she was signed off work with a combination of burnout, depression and anxiety. She couldn't do much more than get up each day, and she couldn't see how things could ever get better.

At the start, Lorien agreed to come in to the gym three times a week. Even if she wasn't feeling sociable or motivated, she resolved to show up and try her best. She had good days and bad days, but with the encouragement of family, friends, and health professionals, she started to see improvements. Eventually, the good days outnumbered the bad.

Lorien returned to work in April 2019 and was promoted a few months later. She knows that her work at the gym – including the support from the

---

trainers and other gym members – was integral to her recovery. She now recognises how important her physical health is in helping to protect her mental health, and that both can be nurtured through exercise in a positive environment.

Tracking wins

The real thing that builds up your confidence? Doing the work required to achieve your goals. And when you track your wins, the payback is even bigger.

When we win, we crave more of the same. We also work best when we have something to focus on and work hard towards, which is why it is so important to track our wins. Simply grinding away for the sake of it isn't much fun, no matter how much good you're doing. And if you're *not* doing anything good for you, then what does it matter?

Too often we chase goals without having full aware-ness of where we are at and what we have achieved so far on our journey – we become too attached to the outcome rather than the process. Will Smith's docu-mentary, *Best Shape of My Life*, where he sets out to lose twenty pounds in twenty weeks, is a great example. He became obsessed, which had a negative effect on the process of achieving his goal. For example, in the first week he trained daily, ate how he was supposed to and still gained some weight. In week 15, having become angry and frustrated by his lack of progress, he gave up altogether. If he had focused on enjoying what he was doing daily and giving himself a little longer to achieve results, he would almost certainly have achieved more and found the results more fulfilling.

As we get closer to a goal, we often move the goal posts and want more. This can be good and keep you hungry for more, but if you do not know where you are at in the process, and if you don't recognise that you are making progress, it can feel like a constant uphill struggle.

We have covered that it is difficult to get started, but the start is the most vital part of any journey. As soon as you've taken the first step on your fitness journey, you'll be in the process of losing weight, enjoying reduced body fat, feeling the way you want to feel, exercising regularly and feeling better in your clothes. You'll also know that your energy and confidence levels are up. Then you'll find other things easier such as meeting new people, and playing with your kids without feeling like you can't keep up.

Life comes at us fast and we are all super-busy, so you must make time for lifestyle changes. It doesn't have to be anything major – it could simply be attending the gym when life gets on top of you, when usually that would be an excuse *not* to go and 'I'll start next Monday'. It could be that you get into a better sleeping pattern or have that awkward conversation at work with a colleague who has been bothering you for a while. You might choose to experiment more with food and find the kids quite enjoy the healthier option, which makes life easier for you too. You might simply become more conscious of the people close to you then arrange a date night with your husband or wife or with one of your kids. It could be something like achieving a personal best in the gym or nailing that big deadline at work. Whatever you are doing and achieving, make sure you note it down so that you fully recognise your progress.

It's worth mentioning here that the number on a set of scales is only one metric, and one we rely on too heavily. I see lots of people at the gym who might not have lost much weight but have a 2–3% decrease in body fat and are down a belt notch or dress size.

It's easy to forget these things when we are busy, but being busy is not a valid excuse. Thinking about this isn't hard – you simply need to create the space and time to think about the things you need to do and get into the habit of doing them. When you do develop those habits, you feel good, and that takes your confidence to another level.

Track your wins to appreciate your growth and personal development, which will boost your confidence and sense of achievement.

Giving is as important here – giving your time and your presence to other people, and doing something without always wanting something back. This will make you feel better about yourself, which is a win in itself. And don't forget to track these wins too.

I am just as passionate about growing, and I track every growth point I achieve.

When your confidence increases, it then increases your thinking, possibilities, and your ability to try new things again. Just like this, would I ever have written a book without writing thousands of emails and doing lots of social media posts since 2014? No.

This book is an obvious win, but it wouldn't have happened without tracking wins – the daily emails and video content that gave me the proof of concept to know a book would be worthwhile, though I did not always feel like doing them at the time.

Just like when trying to get fitter and lead a healthier lifestyle, it's the process that matters. If you don't follow through on the small things, you will not reach that big goal.

It can sometimes be hard to recognise your own wins, but if you look hard enough, you'll find lots of things you wouldn't have done if you weren't making a conscious effort to make progress and stick with the habits that align with your goals. Each and every one of those small things is a win that you can track. Even if you haven't previously tracked wins on your journey, look back now at how far you have come. Think about what you are doing now that you wouldn't have done before getting started. Seeing what you have achieved will improve your confidence. Remember where you were at when you started and how far you have come, without stressing too much on what you haven't yet done or what's next.

This is something I know I need to work hard on. Our business has grown fast and survived a pandemic, but even when things are going well, you can still get bogged down in feeling you are not where you want to be, worrying about what is next and comparing yourself with other people (when you don't really know how or what they are doing).

Whenever you find yourself doing the same, recognise that it isn't serving you well. Take a step back and simply take stock once a week.

Here's the simple but effective process I recommend to all my clients:

Take ten or fifteen minutes on a Sunday to evaluate the week you've just had. Ask yourself what went well, what wasn't as good and whether you did what you set out to. More importantly, track up to three wins in your week. Then consider what you want to get done in the following week. Taking this short amount of time to track your wins will make you more likely to win in the next week, and it will build your confidence. Doing this daily, on a smaller scale through journaling, is also super-powerful.

Now let's look at the bigger picture. Three wins a week comes to more than 150 a year. Tracking those wins gives you concrete proof you are going in the right direction and making progress. If you're journaling daily wins, one win a day is doable, and you will build up an even bigger bank of confidence-boosting achievements.

Whether you do this each week or every day, I guarantee that tracking your wins will make you feel more confident.

TASK: UPPER AND LOWER LIMITS

Grab a pen and paper, think realistically about what you can achieve daily and over a week, and create a personal plan by writing down what an upper-limit day and a lower-limit day look like to you.

It's important you figure out what a day looks like when you get loads done, compared with a day on which you start low but keep aiming to progress a small amount.

The most important thing? You keep showing up and do something rather than stopping or procrastinating. Momentum is critical.

Here's an example of my upper and lower limits:

Upper-limit day

- 45-minute workout
- 10,000 steps
- Calories on point
- 3 litres of water
- 1 big work/business task complete
- Showed up for someone when I didn't need to
- Created some content for social media
- No phone after 7pm
- Bed by 10.30pm

Lower-limit day

- 25-minute workout
- 7,000 steps
- Didn't track calories; ate out but made sure to have extra protein/veg at dinner
- 2 litres of water
- Did what I had to do work wise and dealt with issues I didn't expect
- Bed by 11pm

TASK: ANTICIPATING OBSTACLES

Once you have thought through your typical day, find a quiet spot and write down any obstacles you think may be holding you back and what you would need to do to overcome them.

Here are some personal examples:

- Procrastinating on important work tasks or workouts, when I know I'm less likely to do them later in the day
- Start every day with clearing at least three high-value tasks
- Not having food in the house that aligns with my goals
- Plan each week of meals in advance to ensure I've bought all the necessary food
- Not taking nutritious food into the gym, so I end up grabbing something on the go
- Prepare lunch the night before so it's easy to grab in the morning
- Not planning the next day before I go to sleep, when I know doing that would help me achieve more
- Spend ten minutes each evening planning the next day's times and goals
- Going to bed too late
- Make sure I don't watch TV or use my phone past a set time

Your own obstacles may be related to injury, time, not enjoying what you do – the list is endless.

Simply being aware of your obstacles is the first step in finding the solution. If you overcome any obstacle, it's a win, and that will increase your confidence in overcoming others.

Summary

Confidence is a skill that is earned. Like any reward in life, it doesn't just come to you, but that is where the magic is at. You appreciate it more when you have really seen yourself change and improve.

Confidence won't come out of thin air if you just keep waiting for next Monday. You need to work at increasing your confidence, but it is a skill that can be acquired. Just like doing more repetitions in the gym or attending more sessions, confidence comes through *doing*.

This chapter has covered three straightforward methods for improving your confidence. It is easy to get into the habit of following daily upper and lower limits, anticipating obstacles (and learning how to avoid them) and tracking your wins on a weekly or daily basis. Each of these will help you to improve your mindset and your achievement levels.

Like anything else, these processes may feel awkward or uncomfortable at first, but it will be worth it. Enjoy the wins, set new targets, and keep allowing your confidence to build.

TWO
Character

This chapter is all about the future you – who you want to become. As you read through it, keep the following question in your mind:

What does the best version of you look and feel like?

You are as good or as strong as your character – your character is what you have to fall back on when things go wrong and what gives you internal motivation.

We know where we are at and who we are now – our actions and achievements, our habits, traits, tendencies and thoughts. If you're content with how your life is now, then if it isn't broke, don't fix it. Keep doing what you're doing, looking only for tweaks to improve your life and how you feel.

If you feel you need to make improvements to your life, let's think about how you can make those changes. I want you to future pace and think about your ideal situation and how you would most like to see yourself. Then I want you to simply start acting and thinking that way now.

I have been part of peer mastermind groups for a long time. You take a lot from people who are where you want to be – from how they talk, act, listen and behave. They simply do things differently, and to become different, you also need to think and act differently. It's likely you've heard the saying, 'If you are the smartest person in the room, you are in the wrong room'. It might be good for your ego to be surrounded by less successful or less confident people, but then you simply won't learn as much.

Do what you said you would do

Sounds simple, doesn't it? Just do what you said you would. But how many times do we make promises to ourselves and not follow through on them?

'I'll start next Monday.' (And you never get round to it.)

'I'll wait until I feel fitter.' (You won't feel fitter without working at it.)

'I'll wait until after the holidays.' (Suddenly it's one year later and you still haven't made a start.)

Your integrity and self-confidence grow when you follow through on what you have said you will do, when and how you said you would do it.

Now I want you to make this non-negotiable.

Think first about your daily high-value tasks. Make sure you get those done first, then you can get on with the smaller and easier things. You'll be amazed by the results. It's important to start with the high-value tasks so you don't clutter your day with lower-value tasks, which you know you can do without much thought just so you can say you have been busy. Instead, focus on the things you can do today that will give you real progress.

Set a standard for yourself where you get frustrated if you *do not* do higher-value tasks. Get used to the feeling of going to bed most nights knowing you have made an impact on your own life or on those around you. For example, if you have completed a particularly challenging workout, you will go to bed that night with a feeling of achievement and knowing you have made a difference to your health. And the confidence you feel from that achievement will make you a positive person to be around.

It of course helps to plan ahead, to set goals you know you have to achieve. Your ideal weekly plan might look something like this:

- 3 workouts at specific times

- 8–10,000 steps per day

- Drinking 2 litres of water daily

- Completing that one 'big rock' task at work

- Getting your project finished by Wednesday rather than last minute on Friday

- Writing a social media post to increase your profile or product

Do your best to make this plan non-negotiable. Otherwise, you will almost certainly find yourself looking back at the things you said you would do in the week but didn't get around to, which will make you lose belief in yourself. It will also make it even harder for you to stick to next week's plan.

If I say I'm going to do a workout but don't, or if I say I'll post content on social media and don't get around to it, or if I set a calorie target but exceed it through lack of planning, it seriously annoys the hell out of me. There are of course times you cannot help what happens to prevent you achieving a goal. This isn't about hitting perfection every single day, which is why the plan above doesn't specify days for all the tasks. The only important thing is *progression*.

When you want to get good at something, you're only as strong or as good as your habits.

Where do you think you would be now if you had adopted this mindset five or ten years ago? This question isn't to make you feel bad about what you could have achieved, but to motivate you to achieve as much as you can in the *next* five or ten years.

How much do you think your life and wellness will improve if you just do what you say you will do over the next ninety days?

Remember that you don't need to start with a plan that feels too challenging to be enjoyable or easy to achieve. Make it easy to do to begin with, then slowly build it out. Yes, you'll have days you want to switch off from this level to regenerate and enjoy some downtime. Here's the crucial point, though: be disciplined enough to get back to it when you said you would. If you take only this one thing away from this book, that would be a success for both of us.

CASE STUDY: WILLIAM GARDEN

Willie is a great example of the importance of sticking with a plan. He came to me knowing he had been a lot fitter when he was younger, but offshore life, beer and a lack of routine had got him to a place he wasn't as happy with.

Willie reached out, worked hard and stayed disciplined. After 40 weeks, he had lost more than 6 stone, gained confidence in the gym and changed his mindset to where it should be. Colleagues and family comment on how different he is, and he sees his progress as life-changing. He also says he's still getting new wins every single week.

'I just don't have much willpower or motivation'

This is something I have heard countless times over the years I have worked in the fitness industry, and I get it. It's almost impossible to remain motivated about fitness all of the time. Here's the truth: the same goes for me most of the time, even though this is my profession and all I have done for ten years.

Don't expect to feel fully motivated about fitness, the gym and eating on point all the time, and don't beat yourself up if you don't. Even the people you see who you consider to be super-fit will have days they don't feel like it.

The same goes for the things you get done in life that you know are important. I can guarantee you aren't always hugely motivated to do those either. It's OK to not feel motivated all the time. You aren't weird or in the minority – far from it.

What really motivates us

If you don't control your health, it will control you. It's the same as most things in life. For example, if you don't keep control of your finances, you will pay the price. If you neglect those closer to you, your relationships will reflect the (lack of) work you put into them.

If your husband, wife or kids are only getting the 'dregs' of you because you're too busy to look after yourself, then that needs to change. If you don't protect your energy and mental health, it will own you.

I can't tell you what *should* motivate you – you'll already know that deep down. When it comes to fitness, you may not want to give up some of your free time to work out and for your body to ache for days after. You also likely don't want to have to cut back on the food and drink you enjoy. All these things can be even harder if you have to pay for the pleasure. But sometimes you simply have to resolve to get things done, and you can't wait for motivation to come along and light a fire in you.

Personally, I place a high value on business growth and on family time. To keep improving the business and ensure I don't sacrifice time at home, something has to give. I therefore cut down on drinking, gave up footie and now spend less time with friends. Those are all sacrifices, but they have allowed me to achieve goals I wouldn't otherwise have achieved, which makes me feel better about myself and my life. For me, the payback is worth it.

What challenges our motivation?

When the lease on our first gym was coming to an end and the landlord didn't want to renew, we had no choice but to find a new gym. We had to find something because we had staff to look after, our family's livelihood to protect and more than 100 members who loved coming to our gym. It was a hard six months transitioning to the new place while the other gym was still in operation. We were also expecting our second child but had to throw all our money into the new place.

In a situation like this, you cannot rely on motivation to get you going and move you to the next stage. You simply need to get it done. Sometimes you can't read or talk your way out of pain or towards pleasure – you just have to do the work. Sometimes you need to take uncomfortable action in the short term to get you to where you need to be.

Keeping the end goal in mind is motivational in itself. Would we have ever moved to our current bigger and better premises, in a more central location with more parking, allowing us to have 150 more members and change more lives if we hadn't been forced to? Probably not. But now I am delighted we did it.

Here are just a few examples of daily challenges, which can make it even harder to feel motivated about focusing on our own lifestyle and wellbeing:

- Looking after kids

- Lack of sleep

- Stresses of work or business

- Illness amongst family and friends

Anything like this can get to you and affect your get-up-and-go. It's important to keep your focus, though, on what you really want to achieve. If it means enough to you, you'll get it done. Your actions are a direct reflection of what you prioritise in life and yes, you'll need some help on some – that's only natural.

If you find it hard to get motivated about improving your lifestyle, sometimes it will take something negative like a health scare or a lightbulb moment, when you one day realise you cannot physically do something you used to be able to do. You will then know what means enough to you to motivate you to make changes.

It could be your marriage, or because you want to have kids in the future. You may decide you want to be able to do stuff with your kids/grandkids without being limited by your health or body. You may need an outlet mentally from the stresses of your job because you can feel it taking a toll on your mental health. Maybe your business is consuming your life and you realised that your physical and mental health are affecting your decision making, your general mood with staff and even the future of the business. The pain of staying the same has to outweigh the pain of starting something new and the pain of hard work and change.

Find the trigger for you – the trigger you need to start on and stick to your fitness journey.

What's easy is difficult, and what's difficult is easy

It's easy to do what's convenient. To skip that workout because you don't feel like it. To grab some food on the go or a takeaway or to sit and watch Netflix all night. To say you lack the time rather than looking to *create* the time. To hit snooze rather than getting up early and being active.

By no means are all of these things (and all the other easy or convenient habits) *bad*, but it's vital to know your limits and strike balance. I love Netflix, take-aways and hitting snooze, but I know I can't do those all of the time. It can be easy to be sucked into habits, thoughts or actions that do not serve you well in the longer term, but they will make your life more difficult if you keep doing them.

On the flipside: it can be hard in the short term to do the things that cause more friction – the things that are harder to do but would move you closer to where you want to be. You know that the by-product of sticking to them is that they will make your life easier in the long run – they will give you wins and great results.

The heading of this section, 'What's easy is difficult, and what's difficult is easy,' is inspired by *The Almanack of Naval Ravikant* by Eric Jorgenson. It's a book I highly recommend for learning about mindset, finance and life in general. Naval Ravikant is a smart guy. When you adopt his mindset of choosing difficult over easy, your standards will change, and you will start to feel uneasy about taking the easy option too often.

It is easy to get complacent and fall back into habits that you have worked so hard to conquer. The hard bit is getting back to the difficult options that take a little more willpower. The more you get used to doing that, though, the less you will need to rely on your willpower, and your standards will increase over time.

As your standards increase,
your results improve, and you'll
be on track to achieve your
longer-term goals.

Who do you want to become?

When I was writing this book, I had a call with a coach I was working with at the time, Paul Mort – a successful guy I was looking to learn from. Also on the call was Kevin, who was just getting started in business and wanted to become a personal trainer and, more specifically, a running coach.

Kevin kept saying if or when he got going, and if or when he started creating his programmes, and if or when he got to where he wanted to be. Paul kept coming back to him with, 'You *are* a running coach.'

This is a concept Paul first taught me when I worked with him on a more intense basis in around 2014. I didn't have a gym back then. I didn't even have a very strong personal training business, which is what prompted me to get advice and support from Paul. He called this concept 'acting as if'. Essentially, in your mind you are already where you want to be, and you must act that way – act as if you are already in that position. I didn't then have my own gym or members yet, but I needed to adopt the daily habits of someone who was at that level.

If your mindset and headspace stay where you are now, and you compare yourself only with people at a similar level, you will place limitations on yourself and not reach very far past your current level. To get bigger and better results, you need to think bigger and better. If you aren't where you want to be in terms of health, body shape, mindset, energy or confidence, ask yourself what other people are doing who are at the level you want to reach. Then act as if you are already at that level.

Here are some examples of the questions you can ask yourself when considering people who are at the level you're aiming for:

- How do they think?
- How do they act?
- How quickly do they execute?
- What are their daily habits?
- How do they react to stress?
- How do they set goals?
- What daily actions must I aim for to get to that sort of level?

This can feel intimidating when you start out. There are also limits – I wouldn't look at Elon Musk and wonder why I can't find a way to get to space. I may want to be a great dad, husband and business owner, but I will never try to be Elon Musk. I may want to train a lot, eat well and be as fit and strong as possible, but I am not aspiring to be like Cristiano Ronaldo.

Aspiring to be like certain people and adopting similar character traits and goals is a highly effective method to push you forward, but if you aim too high, there is a danger it could get you down. It's best to take the best bits – those that fit with you and your life – and formulate a combination that works for *you*.

If you are a busy mum with three kids to look after, there's no point comparing yourself with the woman you work with who is twenty years younger, childless and has all the time in the world. If you are a stressed-out business owner, constantly chasing your tail for time and spinning lots of plates, you'll be better off working out three times a week and walking every lunch time instead of aspiring to be like someone who has time to train for two hours every single day.

To an extent, you can only play with the hand you've been dealt. Yes, you must look further ahead and yes, maybe it does sometimes seem unrealistic. But that unrealistic may well propel you further ahead than you had previously deemed possible.

The exciting bit about goals is that they are there to stretch you. Let's think about that person you see at the gym, who you see as super-fit. You may not grow to look exactly like them if you copy their actions over a long time, and let's face it – they probably skip the gym some days, eat chocolate and drink wine like you do. But how often do they do those things? How do they think? How hard do they work? How disciplined are they with their actions? How much of an effort do they make to make daily improvements?

When you know what you want, you need to act as if you are already there.

Who do you want to become? What does an ideal day look like to you? Vision the answers to these questions into reality, and *act*. This stuff works. It can get you down from time to time when you don't feel like you aren't making enough progress, but there's no question this approach has served me far better than *not* doing it.

I surpassed the goals I had back in 2014, when I first spoke to Paul Mort with a hell of a lot of work. It was stressful at times, and I had to give up a lot to get there, including eventually my social life and my football career. It's important to remember that there is always a price to pay for achieving goals.

The same applies to goals I am now thinking about for 2024/2025. I have a board on which I map out things I want to hit in the shorter and longer term. I also remember the goals I set out in April 2020, when we were locked down, including writing a book, moving into our dream home, getting the gym to 250 members, learning about property and starting an online business. Two years on, I have achieved some of those and am working on the others.

Some won't happen. Some will stretch me too far and I may change my mind. For example, one goal on there was to open a second gym, but I no longer want to do that. Most essential: some *will* happen. That's my starting point. It should be yours too.

It is important to live in the here and now, but it's also important to keep an eye on one to three years in the future and slowly build in the habits and mindset that will move you forward to that point. What got you *here* will not always get you *there*.

Continue to evolve your game and your thought processes to move yourself forward to where you want to be.

CASE STUDY: WILLIE GRAY

Willie says that working with us has had an enormously positive effect on his life. Typically, he now gets to the office at 6am, spends an hour on emails and work, then heads to the gym to train. He says this is where his day really starts. Any work stresses are forgotten. Afterwards he feels fully focused, and that stays with him, helping him to feel ready to tackle the day.

We worked with Willie to help him recognise his physical strengths and the areas he needed to spend more time focusing on. We also found out about the injuries he was carrying and his personal goals, then we found ways to help him achieve those goals.

When Willie first came to us, he had had a health scare as well as a knee operation. We devised ways for him to improve his strength and mobility so he could get back to where he wanted to be.

Willie has recently completed a charity challenge, in which he cycled 500 miles over five days. That achievement is testament to his determination to achieve his personal goals.

TASK: CHOOSING DIFFICULT OVER EASY

List three to five daily habits that may be harder in the short term but will make your life easier in the long term.

List five things that motivate you for an all-round better life. Don't just say what you think sounds like the right thing to say; this has to be super-personal to you, i.e. things that genuinely motivate you.

Now write down challenging tasks that will help you to fulfil those five things that motivate you.

Finally, set dates by which you will achieve each of those tasks.

TASK: TOMORROWLAND EXERCISE

Consider this: if you already know how to achieve your three-year goal, maybe it's not stretching you enough.

Grab a coffee and a pen and paper and take 30 minutes to think about all of this.

Be as detailed as possible, writing down as much as you can for this exercise.

This could be about goals for your body, your mindset, your bank account, your relationships and personal life, or what you decide to do for fun and enjoyment (or anything else you want to achieve).

Write an answer to this question: Ideally, how does your life look like three years from now?

Write down any goals that will help you to achieve that.

- Look at those three-year goals and break them down into thirds, i.e. what you need to achieve each year.

- What do you need to achieve within one year to be on track to reach your three-year goal?

- Take your one-year goals and break each one down into the next quarter. What do you need to achieve within 12–13 weeks to be on track to reach each one-year goal?

Write down what needs to be done day to day and week to week to ensure progress has been made for this coming quarter.

Summary

In this chapter we have challenged aspects of your character and your personality traits. At the moment, it's likely that you – like most people – make promises to yourself and don't follow them through. If you simply do those tasks instead of finding excuses, you will achieve a lot more, which will in turn increase your confidence and motivation. You'll also get better results if you choose to work on high-value tasks instead of procrastinating and starting with smaller and easier tasks.

Set yourself a weekly plan and make it non-negotiable. Don't try to rely purely on willpower. Instead, recognise the things that challenge your motivation, and find out what will trigger you to start (and stick to) your fitness journey. It really is as simple as that.

Don't forget, though, that only doing the easy things in life won't allow you to keep improving. Every time you achieve a challenging goal, your standards, confidence and motivation will increase. You need to think big in order to get bigger and better results. You will be amazed by the progress you accomplish simply by making this mindset change and keeping your sights on what you can achieve in the future.

THREE
Clarity

Sometimes life can feel challenging. It's as if you're wading through dirt, and you keep needing to wipe dirt off your goggles – your lens onto life – to see what's around you. You might even have to stop and dig in the dirt sometimes to find ways to flip negatives into positives before you can move forward again. Other days, the lens is clear and you can see clearly out and up into the clouds. On those days, you're not only looking at the here and now but also at how you're moving up and towards your dreams and goals.

It's crucial to set goals and to be clear on what you want to achieve. It's hard to attain goals, though, without learning from negative experiences.

Too often a negative experience can throw you and affect what you want to achieve in the longer term. Sometimes you cannot help that, but often you can instead find a lot of strength from overcoming and learning from a negative experience. This in turn adds new layers to your mindset and your ability to achieve what you want to. Even knowing that you have got through a difficult time can have a positive impact on your confidence levels.

In this chapter we will talk again about how to think differently, but this time in relation to how to find positives in negative situations. We'll also cover some other topics that might surprise you, including the power of being a minority thinker.

Positive focus

Almost without exception, you can find a positive in just about any situation. To state the obvious: bad things happen to us. We all know that. The biggest problem, though? Striving to get through life *without* problems. People genuinely aim for that, but reality dictates it simply will not happen.

You cannot change the fact that
bad things will happen to you,
but you *can* change your perspective
on those things.

For all the wins you've experienced over the years, there will have been a lot of losses. I always wanted to be a football player growing up, and I did get there. Then at twenty-two years old, I was kicked on the soccer scrap heap with no job, no real qualifications or skillsets, and I had to sign on for job benefits (or the dole, as it was called then). That seriously got me down, but I definitely gained a lot from the experience too – it made me grow up and realise what real life was all about, and that nobody cared about my problems. At that time, my problems were a direct reflection of my commitment to football, above everything else, in the previous few years.

I'd gone from living my boyhood dream – being a professional athlete, playing football every day for the team I watched growing up *and* being paid for it. Four days a week I'd been getting to work at 9.30am, having a chat and coffee with mates for an hour, training for two hours, having lunch then going home, before playing a game at the weekend. I got too comfortable in that situation, and then *bang,* it was taken away from me. Suddenly I had no job, no savings and no income, and I had to move back in with my folks, after living independently for a couple of years.

Looking back, I realise now that I didn't enjoy that way of life as much as you might think. It wasn't really as great as it seemed, and there's no question that I prefer what I do now. What we do now changes lives, and it is great to be able to grow a community and interact with people, with no ulterior motive or agenda. Critically, I am also more in control of my own destiny.

At the time, though, it felt like a very negative situation. Still, I looked at the positives and what I was good at. I got a part-time job, working and playing football again, with the late great Neale Cooper. I at least now had some income, which bought me some time to think. I also worked for six months at an electrical chain store. I hated working on the shopfloor so moved to the warehouse, which was real hard work, but I enjoyed working away at my own pace. I knew, though, that I needed to make a change before I got stuck in a rut – I couldn't see myself continuing with that lifestyle for very long.

I therefore got thinking about what I enjoyed most. At the time, personal training was starting to become more mainstream, and I'd always loved going to the gym, so I sold my car – the only real savings I had – and enrolled on a PT course.

That was what really started me on the path to where I am now. I didn't have any real longer-term plans – personal training had really been a shot in the dark – but this still shows how it's possible to turn a negative situation around.

Let's look at a four-step formula that will help you to see the positive in a negative situation.

1. **What** happened – released from full-time football with no savings and no plan

2. **Why** it happened – application wasn't where it needed to be so I wasn't good enough (injury didn't help, but it wasn't the main reason)

3. **The Lesson** – never make that mistake again and double down later in life (what I am doing now)

4. **Apply** – get to work, get qualified as a personal trainer, and get my first clients and proof of concept

Let's relate this to your fitness journey.

A lot of people get put off exercise by a negative experience. Most of our members have been through similar so start with a negative perception of fitness, the gym and personal trainers. We love changing that mindset and getting people to the position where they look forward to going to the gym, enjoying fitness and making it part of their life, to the point they genuinely regret missing any session.

Another example is where a long-standing injury puts people off getting fit. We have had members coming to the gym in real pain. They struggle to get about and move and feel they are a lost cause. Then they learn what they *can* do rather than what they cannot. As soon as they start with us, they can see how this will work for them, which is very rewarding for us too.

Try not to allow one negative experience to put you off for life. Chances are it just wasn't the right time or place. How many times have you had a bad meal at a restaurant? You will still eat out – you just probably won't go back to the same restaurant.

If you have knee issues and keep going for higher-impact workouts, jumping around and/or running, it's unlikely you'll be able to keep that up. Think instead about what you *can* focus on. You could look at your upper body and core, taking the load off your knees but still doing work on your lower body. There will always be a way to work around that niggling, long-standing injury.

If you have your own business and staff, you will have experienced similar situations. There are times when people leave unexpectedly, which hurts, no matter what anyone says. Looking back, though, we realise each time that it happened for the good of the business and the person who has chosen to leave us. Although it takes time and effort to find the right new person, train them your way and embed them in the business, you can bring someone in who is desperate to learn, wants to grow with you and suits your core values. You also learn something new every time you work with someone new.

Whenever the going gets tough, remember that every perfect-looking life, business or person comes with a load of things you can't see. It's like the iceberg analogy – you only see the good, which only makes up a tiny fraction of the whole. You don't see the hard yards, discipline and resilience that brought about the results.

People who get good results also deal well with losses. Ensure you learn and turn short-term negatives into long-term positives.

Don't get too high when you win, and don't get too low when you lose.

CASE STUDY: ANN DARLINGTON

When Ann first came to our gym at the age of sixty-six, she hadn't been able to run for two years due to a knee injury.

Physio and cortisone injections hadn't made any long-term improvement, and Ann felt little motivation to attend the gym regularly.

Shortly after this time, she developed sciatica, which severely restricted her movement. Following advice from her GP, she started trying to strengthen her quads but found it challenging to do this on her own.

All credit to Ann, she was determined to improve this negative situation and started sessions with our trainers, who took time to demonstrate each exercise and offered support and adaptation to ensure success.

Within one month, she was feeling stronger and more confident. Two years on, she now sees the gym as a firm fixture in her life and says she feels stronger than she has for years.

Majority vs minority

There is always gold to be found by following the minority or simply going with your gut instinct. Following the crowd and going with the flow may be the easier option, but you recognise what you deep down need and want. Even if it goes against the norm, sticking to your guns and treading your own path is super-powerful.

You may have a business with a great service or product but find you aren't getting the results you want. Maybe you don't stand out enough.

There must have been times at work where somebody comes in with the home-baked cakes, and everyone keeps saying you should have some. 'Go on ... Live a little ... You don't need to worry about your weight.' Little comments like that don't mean much, but it can still feel hard to hold your own. To get to where you want to, though, you can't always follow the crowd:

'Whenever you find yourself on the side of a majority, it is time to pause and reflect.'
— Mark Twain

If you are doing the same as other people, it makes them feel better about themselves (especially if you're eating cake when they're feeling guilty about it!). It makes them uncomfortable if you are acting and thinking differently.

Take our gym, for example. We could have opened an all-singing, all-dancing gym that was open at all hours, just like most other gyms. We would not have stood a chance because that's already available. We decided instead to be the first gym in our area to start small-group personal training, which was a great hit. Now there are way more options at other gyms, and some have copied or tried to model our success. I'm cool with that. I would rather other gyms were copying us rather than the other way round.

We charge more than other gyms because we decided to deliver a premium level of service, which has enabled us to create a fully successful business. It used to bother me when some people claimed we were too expensive, but I realise now that this is only about a misalignment of values. The same people may drive a fancy car that costs five times more to run than our gym membership, which indicates that they value the car more than what we offer. I use that as an example to demonstrate the value of what we offer. When people consider all the benefits of improving their physical and mental health, their self-confidence and their life in general, they realise that is more important than only looking good in what they drive. I also knew I could never have a team of staff, offering an exceptional service in an innovative and high-quality training environment, if I was charging only £6 per class or gym session. You simply can't get the best for the cheapest prices, and you can't build a truly successful business if you're doing the same as everyone else.

When I first started recording videos for social media, they weren't high quality. I even cringe now when they pop up in my Facebook memories, and at the time my football teammates loved to take the mickey – changing room banter can be brutal. I knew the videos were effective, though; they stood out and drew attention to our business. I laughed and went along with the ribbing from my footie mates, but it didn't bother me. Because I had a longer-term vision for our gym, I knew *why* I was creating those videos. Other people's opinions were not going to pay my bills or feed my kids, and I knew the penny would drop for them a few years down the line. I eventually had to stop playing football and we needed to open a bigger facility because our gym was so busy.

If you deep down know why you are doing something, you don't need to worry about what other people think, even if the results won't materialise for a few years. That is reality.

When I look back now at my football career, I know I shouldn't have followed the crowd as much, especially in having so many nights out when I was younger and only just breaking through. I don't have any regrets now thanks to the direction my life took, but I do admit that following the majority used to hold me back. And like anything else in life, once people think a certain way about you, it is very hard to change that.

I remember one of my coaches at Ross County telling me when I was sixteen, 'People will always judge you, and first impressions are massive.' He was referring to football, saying it's hard to shake a reputation you've made for yourself, no matter how much you change or how hard you try to improve. Whether you're known for being a trustworthy grafter or a lazy party boy, those early impressions stick. Looking now at everyone I knew locally, the ones who went on to big things all had better attitudes right from the start.

That doesn't mean you can never improve, of course – I'm proof of that. I do of course wish in some ways that I had worked harder, listened to other people's encouragement and did as my coaches were telling me. In all honesty, though, I was too worried about what the other players would think; I was young and shy and did not want to draw unwanted attention to myself. I took the easy option, staying under the radar, which caused me bother down the line.

This is a good example of both sections of this chapter. I would have achieved more if I hadn't tried to fit in with the majority. Now, though, I have turned this into a positive – I have learned from this experience and will now always do what I think is best, regardless of what other people think I should be doing. By the time I was starting my new career in the gym game, I had a ruthless attitude about what I wanted to achieve.

It's pretty likely you also worry about what other people will think if you turn down a night out because you want to go to the gym the next morning. Or what people might say if you try a new business idea that fails. Now you need to think 'So what?' You know deep down you'll feel better after an early night and achieving an early-morning gym session.

You'll have failed at something before, and you will inevitably experience some failures in the future. But not taking a risk, avoiding change and trying to do the same as everyone else will probably give you the biggest risk of failure in the future.

People will *always* have opinions – good or bad. You will not change that, and there's no point in always trying to do what other people think is right. What you can do is control the controllable, and that starts with your own thinking – following what you want to do to achieve what you want to achieve.

TASK: POSITIVE FOCUS

List three negative things that happened to you over the past few years.

Now write down what you learned from each of those negative experiences.

Finally, note down what you can take as a positive from each of those experiences. It will likely be something great that's occurred in your life, which simply wouldn't have transpired if the negative thing hadn't happened.

Turning negatives into positives in this way can easily become a life-changing habit, which will have a massively positive impact on your life.

Summary

We all face tough times in life, and I'm sure you've already had to find ways to get past things you have seen as failures. Getting over those setbacks is even easier if you accept from the start that it's OK to make mistakes, and that even bigger failures will serve you well in the long run. It all comes down to perspective.

Beating yourself up about things you haven't done perfectly will only hold you back. Instead, think about the four steps that can help you change the setback into a valuable lesson: think about what went wrong, work out why it happened, learn what you need to do differently next time, then apply this in your life moving forward.

You'll gain the same level of clarity as soon as you decide that you need to do what you know is right instead of following the majority. While modelling and copying other people has some benefits, you will be most successful if you then choose to stand out from the crowd. This is perhaps most obvious in business, where you need to be different to stay competitive in the market. The same goes in just about any area of life, though. As soon as you do what you know is right for you, you will feel better about yourself and achieve more than you ever could if you were only trying to be like everyone else.

PART TWO
METHOD

The mindset element covered in Part One is the groundwork to everything in this book. Now that's in place, we can move on to the method: the coaching, nutrition, lifestyle and habit changes you need to improve your fitness. Remember, though, that mindset is often the most important part of the equation.

Keep all the points from Part One in your mind as you work through the rest of this book – they will help you get the most from all the practical advice and coaching tips we cover next. Having the right mindset will enable you to achieve long-lasting change and to enjoy the whole process.

In this chapter we will cover coaching (and how to get comfortable being uncomfortable), training and workouts, and the lifestyle changes you can make to get the best results. The training itself might not be easy, but then we've already looked at the benefits of choosing difficult over easy.

Gym owners and fitness fanatics are always trying to come up with new gimmicks, meaning there's a lot of rubbish out there. The truth is, though, that the basics will always work and stand the test of time, just as they always have. Instead of inventing new stunts, I will outline clear priorities and make the fitness process as straightforward as possible so that you can see that this really is doable.

If you want to learn the truth about coaching, the importance of accountability, and about what really works to get great results (without arduous, samey workouts), read on.

FOUR

Coaching

There's no getting away from it: in any area of life, coaching will help you to achieve results you simply wouldn't achieve on your own. Whether you're a student, a professional athlete, an employee or a business owner, coaching will help you in areas where you know you need an extra push, and to overcome weaknesses you might not yet have identified.

At the time of writing, I have been a coach for around ten years, which has been extremely rewarding. One of the most important points I have learned in that time is that it takes a lot of work from *both* in the relationship for coaching to yield the best results. A coach can never do the work for you. You have to be willing to put in all the effort your coach demands.

I've been on both sides of the coin. I've found myself in situations where I have wanted results more than the person I am coaching. I also have to admit that I have in the past engaged in coaching programmes where, just by signing up and paying money, I thought I had a given right to something. That is never the case.

That's not to say that all coaching is perfect – far from it. Over ten years of receiving coaching in football, I experienced some good, some bad and some indifferent styles. There is no one-size-fits-all approach – people need different styles of coaching to make them tick. In this chapter I will cover why it is so important to understand that people are all motivated differently, so you must adapt how you coach depending on the situation.

Get comfortable being uncomfortable

Being coached is not always the easiest experience. Let's face it: the point of having a coach is all about being pushed to do what you would not necessarily do on your own, so it can't be about doing what you find easy. It *is* about doing things better, though – a good coach will help you find the optimal way to feel good and achieve more. And you will always squeeze more out of yourself with someone on your case and holding you to account.

There's no denying the benefits of having a coach. Look at top athletes like Michael Jordan and Cristiano Ronaldo, who are the best at their respective sports but still always work with coaches. They know they *need* that extra layer of help and accountability to find the small marginal gains that give them competitive advantage.

You may be a beginner starting out from scratch and need coaching across all areas to make sure you are doing things correctly. You might already be further down the line, at a more expert level, where fine improvements and small gains will make a significant difference to your performance. Whatever stage you are at, coaching will always drive you further forward.

This is the same across the board, regardless of what you are trying to achieve or what area you are working on. Whether you want to improve your fitness, business, weight loss, marketing, mindset, work, life coaching or relationships, if you are committed to doing what's required, a coach will help. You may think you know best, or that you can find out what you need by yourself and go it alone, but the chances are you're only making things easier on yourself rather than confronting underlying issues.

Aim to get to the point where you are comfortable being challenged.

If you think of any big wins or achievements in your life, you will know that the process of getting to that point came down to pure grit. The path to success is never just sunshine and rainbows.

Coaching is tough. If you find that it isn't – if your coach tells you what you want to hear all the time – it's likely you haven't got the best coach. Yes, you need encouragement, but you will make better progress if your coach tells you the truth and what is required.

When I was playing football at a professional level, I hated being told the truth and being slagged off, as it felt to me then. Rather than adopting an 'I'll show them' attitude, I would sometimes try to aggravate my coaches even more, doing the opposite of what they told me to do. Looking back, I now know they were always doing it for my own good, but at the time, it just didn't work for me. Ultimately, I suffered for that because I wasn't open to the coaching and the truth, meaning I didn't get to where I wanted to in football. If there are no fine tweaks or honest conversations, there is no room to grow or learn.

It's important to know that it's okay if you do not click with your coach, you must be patient finding who and what works for you. When I'm coaching, I know who I can help as well as who I won't be able to. I know that I cannot coach a bodybuilder for competition, it's not my strong point, so accept that it's okay to change coach from time to time. Did I not try my hardest at times when I played football? Of course. But would another coach have got more out of me? Possibly. Ultimately, it will come down to you to put the effort in to change, but you must find someone you like and enjoy working with.

I guess that comes down to the coach and you as a person and what makes you tick.

To get the most out of yourself and to ensure you get from point A to point B, you should seriously consider getting yourself a coach. And get used to being uncomfortable – in the long run, this will make you feel much better about yourself.

CASE STUDY: DAVE ALLAN

Dave came to us because he was aware that bad habits were leading to weight gain. He says that, at forty-seven, he'd realised he was on a slippery slope and needed to sort himself out.

Dave was working long hours, spending less time with his family, eating without thinking and drinking too regularly, even though he wasn't drinking to excess. His initial drive was to lose weight, but after a few weeks he saw improvements in all those other areas.

Dave now weighs 2 stone less and is maintaining that weight. He leaves work at 5pm sharp nearly every day, even knocking off early from time to time. He says he feels great – happier, more confident and with bags of energy – and that he hasn't even given

---

anything up. Simply tweaking everything in his life a little, with guidance from our coaches and support from his friends, has enabled him to achieve results he'd never have thought possible.

Dave says that what's surprised him most is that there were no gimmicks. Just receiving sound advice on essential lifestyle changes means he'll be able to live longer and enjoy life much more too.

Sleep and stress management

People can get carried away with trying to find the best workout or the easiest way to burn belly fat, without ever considering two things that affect anything you do day to day: sleep and managing stress.

Better sleep and stress management will improve how you move and fuel your body.

If you don't charge your phone, it just won't work. But are you more bothered about charging your phone rather than recharging your body and mind? Parenting is the first example that comes to mind of the importance of sleep and stress management. If I'm tired and stressed all the time, I simply cannot always be the dad I want to be. I get grouchy and reactive and find myself chasing my tail rather than feeling in control.

The same goes for any other area of life. As a business owner, you will probably act less rationally if you are tired and stressed. Your mind will be foggy, which will affect your decision making, which isn't good for your staff or your customers. If you intend to make it to the gym at 6am every day and you do not have clear boundaries on your sleep, then you will feel too tired and start to skip workouts. You'll then miss the physical or mental benefits, which will make it even more likely over time that you will skip other workouts, creating a downward spiral.

Whatever you are trying to do and whoever you are trying to be, it's safe to say that sleep and stress management are vital.

I know it can be difficult to get enough sleep, especially if you have younger kids. But even if you can't fully control how and when you sleep, it's likely you could improve your environment and your quality of sleep.

Start with small margins to push your boundaries. If you regularly get six hours of sleep, could you push that to seven? Or seven to eight? In terms of environment and quality, focus on preparation. Don't drink too much before bed. Make sure your pillows and mattress are comfortable and up to scratch. It also really does make a difference to stay off electronics for an hour before bedtime to slow your brain down and avoid the negative effects of blue light. Try it for a week to start with and notice the difference it makes to how you feel during the day. I've also found it bad when I read business books before bed, after which I can't sleep while I'm trying to calculate numbers, think of different ideas and write notes when I should be having downtime.

Are there other things you do like this that stop you from switching off? Test what works for you. Some people swear by not eating for one or two hours before bedtime, but I can't do that.

Similarly, you will need to find out what works best for you in managing stress – there is no set way that works for everyone. Personally, I manage stress by working out in the gym and walking. If I don't do one or the other or even both daily, my stress levels increase and I'm not as productive. Rather than being in control of my emotions, I can find them controlling me. If I don't fully control my emotions, I also make poorer decisions as a parent, husband and business owner, as well as for me and my own health.

Some people swear by other techniques such as meditation. If I am totally frank, I can't quite grasp that, but I'm not saying I never will. Keeping physically active does the trick for me, and workouts are the time I can turn off my phone and block out any thoughts that would otherwise be stressing me. By the time I have finished, I have a totally different outlook and perspective, as if I'm seeing things through a different lens.

After a workout I will also have a different level of energy and creativity. That's when I most often write emails and create videos for social media – things I sometimes can't face pre-workout.

I am sure that before the pandemic, the benefits of working out were seen by most people as purely aesthetic. Weight loss, six packs and obsessing about how we look are all still there, but it's fantastic for me to see now that more people get the *real* benefits, especially to mental health. Good health and fitness levels facilitate all the other stuff.

I am convinced that stress management falls into this bracket for every single person, which is paramount in the motivation for all of us to get fit. Stress will *always* be there. I used to long for a stress-free life, but I like to think I have turned a negative into a positive. I now accept that 'good stress' is psychologically positive and that it gives you the push to live your best life. What would I consider to be positive stress? Working hard at higher value tasks; getting out of your comfort zone; a workout and putting your body through stress are just some examples. The reality is you never achieve anything good or worth achieving in life without stress playing a big part.

Whether the stress you are experiencing is good or bad, it can take over when you do not look after yourself and your mindset.

My fat loss priority pyramid

I am sure we all, at some point in our lives, have wanted to lose body fat and look trimmer and leaner. After many years of working in a gym and helping people to lose weight, I know that it is a tough process. The most important first step in that process is accepting there are areas you need to prioritise over others.

People often start out by asking which supplement or protein powder is best to take. Or they focus first on what foods they should be eating or ask us about macronutrients. In reality, those considerations need to come further down the line.

I therefore created the following fat loss priority pyramid, which I include in the beginner's guide for all new members at our gym.

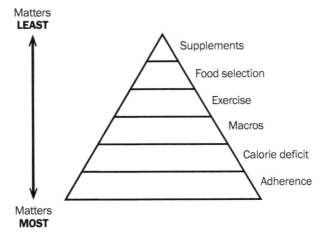

Fat loss priority pyramid

So, let's look at each of the levels in this pyramid, starting with the one that matters most.

Adherence

As covered in Part One, if you start something, you must follow through on what you have said you will do. In a nutshell: be consistent, keep doing what you know you should and stop stopping.

Every time the thought of giving up crosses your mind, think about how tough it was to get started and to get through that initial period. Remembering how far you have already come will help you to keep going. Momentum is key.

Sometimes we are too keen to make progress and overcomplicate things before we even have a routine. You must give yourself enough time to do the simple things first before stepping things up. The discipline of sticking to a plan and making steady progress will help motivate you to keep going. Remember, as we alluded to back in the 'tracking wins' section, motivation and confidence comes primarily from doing the work.

Calorie deficit

Each of us has a basal metabolic rate (BMR). Women's BMR is around 1,500; men's is around 2,000. Essentially, this is how many calories we burn day to day without doing anything 'extra'. For example, even if you have a desk job and don't exercise much, your body still needs energy to breathe and function. You *need* a certain number of calories daily, and this is where the old 'eat less and do more' saying is a bit backwards. You do more and more, eat less, burn out and become disillusioned with the whole process and end up back at square one. Yes, you need to create a calorie deficit in order to lose weight but there's a balance to strike here.

The BMR gives us a guide to work from. If we want to lose weight or body fat, we must maintain a small or large calorie deficit. This needs to depend on what you can do, stick to and enjoy, without resorting to self-sabotage or stopping. It's worth noting that the opposite applies if you are training to gain muscle – you have to eat more to ensure you do not drop into calorie deficit.

You can create calorie deficit by tracking calories. Use an app such as MyFitnessPal and input your food intake – honestly and daily – to increase your understanding and accountability. You don't need to do this forever – even only a week or two can help you understand how much you consume and how much you need to cut down. The goal here is not to make you obsessed with calorie counting or reliant on apps. It is to give you the tools and knowledge you need to be self-sufficient. Once you understand what your body needs, you won't normally need to use apps, apart from times you want to reset or remind yourself.

Macronutrients

Macros are the nutrients we need for energy, made up of fat, protein and carbohydrate. Most people who come to our gym wanting to lose weight or body fat don't fully understand the importance of the ratio of the different macronutrients, and it's vital to strike the right balance.

For fat loss and toning up, protein is the most important macro we need, and people generally struggle to eat sufficient quantities. Protein intake is critical because you *do not* want to lose weight *and* muscle mass. Losing muscle mass makes it harder to decrease body fat and to achieve the aesthetic look you desire. Often, when people achieve serious weight loss via slimming clubs and heavily restrictive diets, muscle tissue is wasting away. This is not healthy in the longer term, especially because it becomes much harder to build that muscle back up again.

You need to ensure you consume 1.5–2 grams of protein daily for every kilogram of your body weight. For example, an 80 kg male should be aiming for 120–160 g protein daily.

Carbohydrates get a bad reputation, but you *need* them. Your energy, your mood, your performance during workouts and your general enjoyment of food depend a lot on carbs. Generally, you may just need to reduce your carbohydrate levels; some people see amazing results simply by cutting out their main carb source, which is often bread. It's unlikely you will burn enough energy to justify the quantity of high-carb foods you are currently consuming.

Vegetables are vital in any diet for their fibre and all the other nutrients, which keep the standard of your diet high. You can eat a high volume of vegetables, which makes you feel full (so craving less food), and you don't need to worry about the calories they contain.

To ensure I am eating enough vegetables and staying fuller for longer, I always keep mini bags of mixed veggies in the freezer. Try eating a bag or two a day and see if you crave as much other food. I bet you won't.

Exercise

The next step in losing weight or body fat is exercise, whether via intense workouts, strength training, steadier cardio exercise or a general increase in movement. You can track the amount of calories you burn using a smartwatch or gym heartrate monitors, for example. One thing to remember is these will only give you a rough guide – both have a margin for error (up to 10–15% either way). Watches and heartrate monitors therefore aren't fully reliable, although both can encourage healthy habits, helping you to create a calorie deficit through your exercise.

If you are female and burn roughly 250–300 calories through walking or going to the gym every day, if you also drop your daily calorie intake to 1,300/1,400, you will create a 300–400 daily deficit. If you do this five days out of seven and are slightly more relaxed with food on the other two days, you will have a solid deficit over the week.

The same goes for men, adding only roughly 500 to the daily calorie intake. The opposite applies if you're looking to gain muscle mass or weight. Instead of a deficit, you would be looking for a calorie surplus, gradually increasing calories in your diet.

There are two important things to note here. If you are making a real effort with your diet or tracking your calories, you do have to do it seven days a week, including weekends. Having the odd beer or glass of wine is fine, but drinking more than that every weekend, compounded by a couple of takeaways, could completely sabotage the work you have put in throughout the week. I am sure we have all been there, planning to 'be good' this week, starting the week well and managing to keep up with exercise and a strict diet from Monday to Friday. Then as soon as you get to Friday evening, your mindset goes from one extreme to another, and you forget about all your best intentions until Monday (or never get back to them at all).

It is important to relax and enjoy life, but if you really want results, your actions must align with your goals 80–90% of the time. If you really can't do that, you might need to be more realistic with your goals.

Even if your calories are on point over a set period, it takes time, discipline and consistent tracking of habits to get results.

Don't aim to be in deficit for too long. A good pattern is to maintain your calorie deficit for four to six weeks maximum then move on to a calorie-maintenance phase. In maintenance phases your performance and energy should be higher since you're eating slightly more daily, enabling you to tackle other targets. Ultimately, do what you can and only what you're happy with. You must approach it in a way that best suits you. You may just like exercising and have an awareness of what you're eating without worrying about deficits. You may find there are times you want to see and feel change, perhaps at a certain time of year or in the run up to an event. Just know that you won't always be able to maintain a deficit all year round. This is something we will cover later with our Traffic Light System.

Food selection

In short: keep your diet rich in terms of quality and nutrients.

Stick to a calorie deficit, but make sure you also don't fill your diet with junk. For example, if you know you will get results from 1,500 calories per day, that doesn't mean you can eat 1,500 calories of processed foods, including a takeaway pizza for dinner.

Stick to a healthy split and balance. 80–90% of the time, try your best to reach your calorie target with a good balance of protein, veggies, fats and carbs.

Allowing a treat or a cheat meal to make up the remaining 10–20% won't do much harm. It will also likely help you to adhere longer term to your plan if you don't completely eliminate the food or drink you enjoy most.

Supplements

It is easy to see supplements as a magical weight-loss elixir. But things like protein powders won't give you miracle results, and they are not a meal replacement as such.

If you have carefully followed all the other steps above, then it may well help you to supplement your diet. It's good to have protein powder handy for days you're looking to get some extra protein in or to recover post-workout. Creatine supplements supply energy to cells, particularly to muscle cells, so they can aid your performance in the gym and help you to reach your goals more quickly. Vitamin D is great, especially because most of us probably don't get enough daily sunlight. I don't generally recommend supplementing your diet in other ways.

Training

Recently, one day around Christmas time, the weather was very cold and the roads icy. As I left the house on my way to the gym, I took an absolute flyer. I ended up with both feet in the air, convinced in the split second I was falling that I was going to crack my head or break a bone. Fortunately, my arm hit the step before my head did, so my forearm took most of the impact, but I still think I was lucky not to suffer a break. There's no doubt in my mind, though, that my diet and all my training also helped me, which brings me to two important points.

Strong bones

Including plenty of calcium in your diet is of course crucial, but it's also unquestionable that physical activity and strength training lead to stronger bone density. Not only that, but improved fitness helps with our physical balance and coordination, reducing the chances we'll suffer a fall in the first place.

Our risk of falling increases as we get older. But if you commit to workouts and strength training, you give yourself the best chances of avoiding a fall, and of reducing the damage if you do.

Why and how we design our fitness programmes

At DM Elite we put a lot of time and thought into designing the ideal programmes for all our members. Over time, through training myself and helping lots of clients, and having been in the industry for over ten years, I have found a 'sweet spot' – a template for the ideal fitness programme that covers all bases.

My template is made up of eight workouts. With seven days in a week, you might be wondering how we fit these in. Stick with me and I'll explain.

1. **Strength work**

    - Target: 3 times per week

    - 8–10 hard strength sets across big muscle groups, over 2 or 3 sessions

    Keep this up and your shape will continue to improve. And it just feels good.

2. **High intensity training (HIIT)**

    – Target: 2 times per week

    – Should never need to exceed 20–30 minutes actual work if done correctly

We are really testing our heart rate here. Things like heartrate monitors or smartwatches are great if you really want to delve into the data. Essentially, HIIT is about working hard for short, intense bursts, separated by small rest periods. Frequently completing high-intensity HIIT training is great and can make you feel great, but you have to be careful not to overdo it, to avoid injury and fatigue.

3. **Steady cardio**

    – Target: 2 times per week

    – 40-60 minutes per session

This is probably the easiest training to do on your own, and you can achieve one hour per day with a decently paced walk. Alternatively, you could maintain a heartbeat level of between 130 and 150 beats per minute on the bike or rower, working at about 60–70% of your maximum.

Steady cardio can be part of a recovery day. It's important this element of cardio is light and done as an active recovery, rather than a workout. This is a seriously undervalued tool in your health armoury and is fantastic for your long-term health. Remember: harder doesn't always mean better.

4. **Speed/power work**

   - Target: 1 time per week

   Speed is essential to this type of workout – you must keep doing things fast. That doesn't mean you have to do sprints: in the gym, it could be rope work, fast feet, ladder work, ball slams, etc.

   As we get older, we don't necessarily lose strength – we lose power. This type of workout is great for things like falls. Your reaction time, coordination and ability to move quickly will improve if you do this regularly. Doing speed/power work once every week is crucial to your power output and can help you remain injury free.

You could cover all eight of these workouts over four or five days. Do your speed work at the end of a strength session. Add some HIIT work at the end of a strength session. Get outside and walk for an hour on a rest day.

Don't worry about getting all of these workouts in every single week. You need to factor this in with how often you can and want to make it to the gym. But if you're not really doing much now, and you switch to going to the gym only twice a week for a year, it will still make a big difference to your overall health. And hopefully, as your confidence and fitness improve, you will find ways to increase your number of workouts.

CASE STUDY: NOME WILL

Nome came to us because he wanted to lose weight. He weighed in at around 19.5 stone and knew something had to change.

Nome admitted that making that initial contact and the fear of the unknown were his biggest obstacles, but it helped him to run through the programme on the phone with us. We made everything as clear as possible, and it was great when he started a programme with us soon after.

As the programme progressed, Nome became increasingly aware of how it affected other areas of his life such as balance and goal setting. Nine months in, he is now happy with his new weight of 15 stone 6 lb, and he now wants to keep fit and maintain the routine of the programme. He says he now recommends our programme to anyone looking for a positive change in life.

TASK: YOUR OWN FAT LOSS PRIORITY PYRAMID

Look again at the pyramid below and work out what you most need to focus on now.

Have you managed to train your mindset, using the methods from Part One, to ensure you will be able to adhere to any plan you create?

If you are sure you have that level of commitment, work out your ideal calorie deficit then use an app to start tracking your calories. Tweak your diet as required, taking each week into account rather than only being happy if you keep within your calorie limit for one or two days.

Remember your macros – it's vital you consume enough protein to prevent muscle loss, whilst not eliminating carbs altogether.

While exercise isn't the most important level in the pyramid, as many people think at first when they are trying to lose weight, it's still important that you ensure you are moving enough to burn calories and strengthen muscle. Try using a smartwatch or heartrate monitor to gauge the effectiveness of your exercise.

If you have covered all four base levels of the food pyramid, make sure you're also eating enough high-quality food, including the nutrients you need to keep yourself healthy.

Finally, only when you are happy you are fulfilling all the other requirements in the fat loss priority pyramid, you may choose to supplement your diet with carefully selected supplements.

Summary

Coaching isn't easy, and you may at times feel like you hate your coach, but I can just about promise that you will still love what they get out of you. A good coach will give you the knowledge, expertise and account-ability you need to get to the next stage. They will guide you in the right direction, making sure you do everything you need for your own long-term good. Remember that you chose to be coached for a reason, so you need to trust the process, which in time will lead to good habits.

Essential to losing weight and body fat are sleep and stress management. These are not the most obvious factors, but you will reap the rewards when you find ways to get more sleep and avoid or cope with stress.

After that, it's important to focus on the different fac-tors of weight loss, as illustrated in my fat loss priority pyramid. Build each layer in before you move on to the next one, making sure you don't jump ahead and complicate things when you don't need to.

Finding ways to build regular training into your life-style is vital to your health in more ways than one, not least in improving your bone density, balance and coordination. Your weight and overall health will improve, especially if you stick with the workout tem-plate I have outlined in this chapter.

FIVE

Community and environment

Whether you're eating out at a particular restaurant, returning to a gym or going to your local for a beer, there are two main things that will keep you going back to the same place: environment and community.

We are social creatures. Once we feel safe in an environment that meets our needs, we will keep coming back if the community is strong. We value our experiences with people above all else.

With DM Elite, I was determined to provide a high-quality environment. More importantly, I wanted to create a strong community of like-minded people, who all become friends and enjoy working at getting fitter and stronger *together*. Yes, people join gyms to get stronger, to get fitter and to lose weight or body fat. But there is little motivation to *keep* attending a gym without the people, the events and the camaraderie, and knowing that people at the gym care for you and your progress.

A community is a group of people who work and grow together.

If you have a friend who wants to achieve a similar goal, and they are more motivated than you, it will doubtlessly help you to keep on track. If you are in that session and feel like slowing down, but other people are there driving you on, it will help you to keep going.

The power of accountability

Accountability can be used in many ways, for example if you have a coach who checks in on you once a month outside of workouts to ensure you are on the right track. Accountability from your peers is also hugely powerful. Even as a gym owner who has been in the fitness industry for ten years, I still need to keep myself accountable, so I make sure I get some of the staff at the gym to train me. I put my name down for a specific time, which I then know I need to stick to, and I have fewer distractions when I am working with the others. I could do the same workout on my own, but then I'm not as engaged, working at my own pace and more likely to take breaks to check my phone. Having an extra layer of accountability always helps.

They say you are the average of the five people you spend time or hang out with most, which is why I try and be involved in groups of people who are ahead of where I want to be. The more time I spend with them and hear about what they are doing, the more likely I am to get closer to where they're at.

If you always meet friends at the bar, the chances are you'll drink more. If you spend time scrolling negative news on Facebook, your energy will reciprocate that. Alternatively, if you meet up with people you like at the gym, there's no question you will work harder and enjoy getting fitter together.

I can't emphasise highly enough or too often the importance of having expert guidance from a coach. The coach will have experience of helping other people just like you, and that extra layer of help and accountability will ultimately save you a fortune in time and stress (and money, if you have coaching in your business or career).

It is possible to go it alone, but let's be honest – that is lonely. I don't really gain new knowledge or secrets from the gym owners' business group I am now part of – it is just good to have support when I really need it. It keeps me on the straight and narrow and helps me avoid big mistakes. Within one of these groups, we would meet at a certain point – discuss challenges, ideas, and targets for the next meet up. In between those time frames generally you would check in with everyone once per week and by the time the next meeting comes, you're focused to achieve what you set out to because we held ourselves accountable to these goals in the previous meeting.

When it comes to workouts in the gym, I of course know what I am doing – it's my day job. When I'm on my own at the gym, I will still go through the motions, but it's never the same. I much prefer to get some of my staff to coach me, and I join the small-group sessions with members. That pushes me more than I would achieve on my own.

If you think you push yourself to your maximum capacity *without* a coach, then I'm afraid you might be lying to yourself. The longer you get into the process, it is the tiny gains and coaching points that only a coach can see that can move you to the next level.

In the past, I went to a gym owner who is experienced and had made a lot of expensive mistakes. He offers a mentoring programme that costs £500 per month. That may sound super-expensive, and it is a chunky investment, but let's look at it this way: one mistake can bury your business and your livelihood. This gym owner has probably lost money and time on mistakes in staffing issues, understanding business metrics, gym layout, overall capacity and pricing, and he can tell other gym owners about what they need to do to avoid the same, and what they should be thinking about up to three years down the line. I therefore see the cost of his programme as a sound investment.

Personal trainers are also a fair investment, but what price can you put on your energy, fitness, confidence and all-round mood increasing, and being able to do things you couldn't do before? The same people who complain about the cost of personal trainers likely spend more on nights out, booze and the latest phone models.

Coaching can be seen as expensive … or the best value you will ever get. I guess this comes down to your mindset and perspective. If I know a person is going to get more out of me than I would on my own, it makes more sense to me to do that rather than spend £1,000 on a pair of trainers.

Customer experience

The goal of this section is to help you find your DM Elite. If you live local to Inverness and are NOT coming to us, then please reach out. We would love to show you what we are all about. But if you're further afield I would love for you to find something that works for you. This is something I am super-passionate about, and I never take our gym members for granted. Lots of businesses strive for customer satisfaction, and I'm sure you have been asked to complete any number of satisfaction surveys. They hardly light you up inside, though, do they?

I love learning new customer experience tricks by observing other businesses outside of the fitness industry – hotels, restaurants, hair salons, etc. I even visited New York to see what was being done elsewhere and to gain ideas for our gym here in Inverness.

Like most people, I've done business with different places over the years and experienced some sloppy customer service. For instance, they don't remember stuff about you (even your name), you are treated like a number and not a person, it takes ages to get a reply when you contact them, and you get passed around between different departments. Then when you do get hold of the person who should help you, they seem to feel they are doing you a favour, and your issues aren't dealt with efficiently.

In my experience, few places go above and beyond and aim to *wow* you. That has always been my goal here both at the gym and with the people I coach online. You don't deserve to put up with lousy service – choose businesses that go above and beyond to make you feel valued.

We may have upwards of 250 members, but I know everyone's name, and I emphasise the importance of that to all my staff. Just like motivation to get fit, being busy isn't an excuse – we can never get complacent on customer service. Every one of our team knows I want them to do all they can for our members to give them the best results possible in an environment they value and enjoy coming to. I must admit, it gets difficult to maintain the same standards as your business expands, but I like the challenge. We are bigger than we were in 2016, but in my opinion, we are ten times better.

We make sessions fun, effective, varied and enjoyable. Some trainers may see more importance in repetition, but most people will get bored. We want our members to keep enjoying training rather than finding it a chore.

It often happens that a new member is anxious, having never done any gym work before. I love then seeing two or three months later how they love the gym and cannot get enough of it. This is why we focus on helping other people enjoy using DM Elite. It's also the reason for our tagline: 'The gym for people that don't like gyms.'

When we think about gyms, we might well picture people hogging the free weights area, dropping big weights and grunting, with other people posing, more focused on how they look. We likely imagine lots of mirrors and busy classes that are booked out at peak times. We think of twelve-month contracts you can't get out of, even if you never show up. It's less likely you'd think immediately of *community*.

Before we opened our own, I always thought of gyms as soulless places. I never used to like training in conventional gyms, and in the five or six years I was a personal trainer without my own gym, I *never* worked in a gym. I just knew they weren't for me. When we thought about opening our own, we knew we had to create something different.

Remember that thing about following the majority or the minority? We focused on the members and building a safe, inclusive environment that people enjoyed coming to and where they made friends – those were priorities from the get-go. We don't have mirrors, which may seem a small thing, but our members love it. We never focused on scale weight or measured members' progress based on that.

We made our training unique from the very start. We put a big emphasis on events outside of the gym so members get to know one another better. When we hire trainers, we don't look only at how good a coach they are or could be – we look at the person and whether they fit our core values. Lifestyle change has always been a bigger focus for us than short-term transformations.

We also make sure our members can book what they want, where capacity isn't an issue. Most gyms are designed for 90% of the membership base to fail and not show up. That is no use in our own business perspective because we don't tie people in to contracts, and no one would pay us in excess of £100 a month to not turn up. Commercial gyms can have membership bases upwards of 4,000. There is no way they could serve all those people if they all wanted to turn up – it would be a health and safety hazard and not enjoyable for the customer. We have an overall capacity at which we can maintain our standards, and we know our limits.

If you do not like gyms, that's cool; there are other options out there for you. Don't hesitate to reach out to us at www.dmelite.co.uk to see what we can do for you.

CASE STUDY: STANLEY BROWNE

Stanley says he is 'not a gym person'. He'd never liked gyms, preferring instead to improve his fitness through group sports. However, he was impressed by a video about DM Elite so signed up for a session.

The first thing Stanley noticed at our gym was the lack of mirrors, which he felt removed the 'all about me and how I look' syndrome. He found our instructors welcoming and friendly, and he liked the simple and effective layout of our gym.

Above all, he liked that other gym members came from all walks of life, all with different levels of fitness. He immediately noticed a community spirit,

---

> with people gently encouraging each other verbally, or just with a nod of acknowledgement.
>
> Stanley says that it feels more like a community hub than a gym, and that this motivates him more than anything to remain a member and to keep attending sessions.

Summary

In this chapter we have looked at how our environment and the people around us play a significant part in motivating us to improving our lifestyles. It's vital that you feel comfortable and safe in your gym so that you want to keep going back. Even more important is the people you train with. Motivation and results will get you started, but being part of a positive community will keep you going.

It's also crucial to remember the power of accountability in helping you to remain motivated to improve your fitness. Whether it's your coach or other gym members who are reminding you of your goals, there's no doubt that you will achieve more than if you were answerable only to yourself. You are the average of the five people you spend the most time around, and it is vital to have role models that you can look up to and gain advice and wisdom from. If you want to be fitter, spend time around people who value fitness.

Finally, customer service might not be the first thing you think of when it comes to gyms, but it's vital that you feel valued, welcome and safe in your environment. Whichever gym you consider joining, make sure that the customer experience is one of the managers' main priorities. Knowing that your gym appreciates you will make a big difference to your motivation to stick to your fitness plan.

PART THREE
MOMENTUM

Your long-term results will be nothing without momentum. Stopping and starting repeatedly is an easy trap to fall into, but over time it gets harder and harder to get going every time you aim to start afresh.

I'm sure you have heard the saying that life is a marathon and not a sprint, and this saying is particularly true in relation to your fitness journey. Slow and steady wins the race.

There are of course times in life when you need to get somewhere fast, but in fitness it is vital to focus on longevity. It always takes time to achieve and maintain weight loss, and to build your strength and fitness levels, so there's no point in trying to find a quick fix.

In this final part of the book, we will look at the motivation you need to start on your fitness journey and how you can get the best results through steady and carefully planned progress. We will also consider the power of consistency and how you can achieve that in your training schedule. Mindset is as critical here as in any other part of your journey. As your results change and improve, so must your thinking.

SIX

Change

Change only happens when the pain of staying the same outweighs the pain of change.

Generally, people do not like change. When we moved our gym's location, we had to hire new staff and charge higher prices than other gyms, and a lot of our members weren't too happy about the situation at first. The positive effect of moving was a bigger facility though, so we could provide more value to the member, better parking, more changing space and a 'community space' upstairs which allowed people to get to know each other outside the sessions.

Things will only happen when the change means enough to the people involved. If you resist change when you need it, you will also be resisting progress. I therefore always look to move things forward to stay in the game. *Not* looking forward doesn't excite me.

People have even said I can be too ready to take risks, by doing new stuff and always looking to move the business forward. I disagree. For me, the riskiest thing you can do is do nothing at all, simply standing still and accepting where you are.

There will of course be challenges. If you want to lose weight, for example, it's going to be tough at times. Giving up your free time to put yourself through pain (at the start), while giving up some of your favourite food and maybe even paying for the pleasure of it all ... but the benefits will far outweigh any of the drawbacks.

Considering the alternative outcome should give you the motivation you need to change. If you consider that you may not live as long if you don't get fitter, or you may not be able to move as freely, or you may not have the energy to play with your kids or grandkids, that will hurt a little. It is likely that the pain of facing those adverse outcomes will encourage you to take the first step. If these points don't mean enough to you, you probably won't be motivated.

Don't do nothing, simply blaming a lack of willpower. Find the pain you need to give you motivation. Find that why, then achieve what you want to achieve.

I am terrified of losing my fitness and getting out of shape. I do not want to use the business, young kids or 'being busy' as an excuse.

I fear losing our business and everything we have worked so hard for. That's why we put our all into doing what we do every day and ensure we are always doing all we can to improve. If you stay still in today's world, you will be passed by.

As much as I want that success, I fear getting to a point where I don't see my two girls as much. Fortunately, that is not the case, and we spend lots of time together.

Getting 1% better

Progress beats perfection. Progress is achievable, but striving for perfection is setting yourself up for failure.

The word 'kaizen' is Japanese for 'change for better', referring to any level of improvement. Kaizen is also the name of the Japanese concept of continuous improvement of working practices, personal efficiency, etc – improvement in any area of life.

Things don't happen overnight. Small changes – even only 1% at a time – and maintaining momentum over a long period yield the best results.

Usually, people start out with high levels of motivation, which can lead to big steps in short periods of time. This is helpful for urgent and short-term goals, but it can be detrimental if you are looking to change long-term habits and your all-round lifestyle.

There is no point in committing to something you can't see yourself doing for a decent length of time. You are likely to burn out or face injury – or experience other adverse effects – because things aren't going at the correct pace. When people join our gym, no matter where they are on their journey or what they want to achieve, they start with our 28-Day Challenge. That comprises ten sessions rather than twenty for a reason, and we don't enforce strict nutrition changes at this point. I want us to keep our members accountable and enable them to achieve their goals, but I also want them to enjoy the whole process. It's always more effective to be process-focused rather than results-focused … and the by-product of an enjoyable process is *results*.

DM Elite is all about getting 1% better over a specific period, which is a concept people can struggle with at first. But if you get 1% better every week, that's 52% better in a year. If you could improve a habit within one year, if it didn't feel like it was a huge chore and it happened seamlessly, you would no doubt be delighted.

One example of this is Jerry Seinfeld, well known for his 'don't break the chain' strategy. As an up-and-coming comedian, he set himself the goal to write one joke a day, every single day without fail. That wasn't a huge goal in itself, but he knew that over time it would compound to the point he had an endless supply of jokes.

Similarly, when I started on this book, I knew I needed to write 30,000 words within twelve weeks, so I broke it down: 3,000 words a week, with six writing days a week, so 500 words a day. That felt much more manageable, and once I got started with writing, everything else flowed. Although I am passionate about the topic and it meant enough to me to write this book. I knew from the very start, that I wouldn't be able to write it in one go, so I broke it into chunks.

You may not think that any of the following may change your life:

1. 7,000 steps a day

2. 2–3 litres of water a day

3. A 30-minute workout a day

4. Cutting back on snacking or liquid calories

There's no doubt, though, that each of these will make a big difference when compounded over weeks and months. The key is not to give up.

Joe Wicks is hugely famous now but when he started, nobody liked or commented on his social media content. He kept going, though, posting multiple times a week until he gained trust and impact. Having started a business or launched an idea on social media people can be too quick to take down a post if it does not get enough likes. If Joe Wicks had given up like that, he would not have become the huge hit he is now.

The same goes for your life goals and your fitness aspirations. Know what to do, why you are doing it and just keep persevering. Even if there is a gratification delay (which is something I cover later in the book), you will eventually enjoy great results.

CASE STUDY: MUIR MORTON

I first met Muir when he coached me while he was playing for Ross County U15/17 football teams.

During his late twenties and early thirties, Muir met and married his wife, and they started a family, which made remaining active much harder. He was facing other challenges too. Both his parents had experienced health scares, and Muir knew of a long line of hereditary illness in his family. In 2018 he was the heaviest he had ever been, tipping the scales at just over 14 stone. He was also finding it difficult, with work and a young family, to manage his time.

Muir knew that he had lost some of his motivation and capacity to train, and he realised something had to change. Above all, he says that he wants to be able to enjoy being active with his children for as long as he possibly can.

He got back in touch when he noticed our 28-Day Challenge on Facebook. He had only planned to use the 28 days to kickstart himself into his own training again, but three years later he is still an active member of our gym.

Muir says that our gym, staff and sessions have undoubtedly helped him on his health journey – he's lost just over 10 kg in weight and regained a real focus about his own personal fitness. This has had a positive impact on his professional and personal life. He has more energy at work and more time to spend with his children. He also finds it easier to complete tasks and solve problems, and he says he feels more assured and content on the days he has trained. Even his golf game has improved, and he now finds himself continually looking for more challenges, from hill walking to applying for promotion.

Athlete vs amateur mindset

I love the athlete mindset, and you do not have to be an athlete to adopt it. It relates to the topic on aspiring to be like certain people, which I covered in Part One.

This is about acting as if you are a top athlete. These guys get all the glory and headlines, but nobody sees how resilient they are or the work that goes into being a top athlete. The goal is to adopt the mindset of an athlete instead of the mindset of an amateur. The athlete gets the job done, no matter what.

Cristiano Ronaldo is now one of the best football players ever, but he wasn't always. He had the athlete's mindset before he made it big, and since then he has had to work even harder on that mindset to stay at the top.

Sometimes you can lose a bit of weight and get fitter specifically for an event or holiday … and then down tools. You can get complacent and undo all that hard work you put in over a long period, which is giving your future self a lot of work. Rather than yoyoing up and down, adopt the athlete mindset and work hard to create new goals. Now you have hit that weight-loss goal, can you now focus on another event or set a different performance-related goal?

You never complete fitness or life in general. There are always new ways to improve, innovate and grow further. I don't think anyone that loves fitness and knows they are super-fit or a very successful businessperson ever thinks they have 'completed it' and can rest on that. That drive that got them there will always look for new ways to better themselves. There should always be new opportunities that your fitness and health can propel yourself towards. The most successful people find ways to motivate themselves and keep getting better. In the series *The Last Dance*, Michael Jordan famously makes stuff up in his own mind to motivate himself and light a fire in order to be able to succeed.

Olympic athletes that run the 100-metre sprint, for example, train multiple times a day for many years with little recognition. They are training for a ten-second race that they may not even qualify for. If they do qualify, they might get disqualified or be one hundredth of a second behind the gold medallist and walk away feeling defeated. Think how much they must use their athlete mindset to pull them through all those years of training.

Next time you feel too tired or you've had a tough day, ask yourself, 'What would he/she do?' and 'How would they think?' You can get the work done, regardless of how you feel.

Two teams can play for ninety minutes at the same sort of intensity and the team that loses is exhausted without an ounce of energy left. The team that wins feels on top of the world and ready to play again.

You don't have to be smashing it, exceeding your goals every day. You only need to have an awareness of and focus on your progress. That will allow you to achieve wins, and winning builds momentum. Winning also breeds confidence and energy, which is why it's so vital you track your wins.

To win, you need to be your own inner athlete. You may not be Ronaldo, but you do attend the gym, and you do want to get fitter and stronger, so you are already an athlete. Now you only need to create the mindset from *within* that you are a top athlete.

This new mindset will also help you to see obstacles as opportunities. I always think as a parent that if I use excuses to not do something through laziness, fear or lack of motivation, then my children may grow up and think it's OK too. Kids model your actions and what you say. Aimee and I are big on setting an example to the girls. Our daughters know we train at the gym four or five days a week. They see how hard we work on our business in the evening, and they will understand in time why we did that. Sometimes we find it hard to get our work/life balance perfect, but sometimes needs must.

You may not want to go to a workout because you are too stressed, but you could decide to see it as an opportunity to relieve stress and forget the day that has passed or the things that are keeping you awake at night. It can give you a chance to detach and focus on 'you time.'

As a parent, making it to that workout is a chance for me to teach my kids that it's important to look after your health – more important than the reasons *not* to do it.

For me, that workout is also a chance to think creatively – it releases space in my mind. When writing this book, a workout always generally preceded a writing session.

Avoiding complexity

When you are trying to build momentum, one of the silent killers can be information overload. This is also known as information paralysis, where you have too many decisions to make or too much to think about a topic, to the point where you do nothing about it.

I have experienced this myself by following too many business mentors or motivational speaker types. They are all successful and make great points, but there can be too much for anyone to take in. They often give conflicting advice – one influencer says hustle until you drop, while the other promotes balance. Somebody says go high fat / low carb, while another preaches the carnivore diet. Multiple physios may give you completely different prognoses and rehabilitation drills. Similarly, personal trainers all have different styles. You just need to work out what works for *you*, go with one method and trust the process.

One thing is for sure: the basics will stand the test of time.

With health, fitness and weight loss, people are quick to jump on new trends. New strategies or the latest fad will give you an initial buzz in the short term, but that will wear off in time … and the cycle continues. There is then the danger that people will blame the process itself instead of admitting that they haven't put the work in. You will achieve much better results if you stick with the basics, keep it simple and commit to gradually making progress. Trust the process and give it time – this alone will change the game for you if you don't overcomplicate things.

Don't listen to people who are trend hoppers. They will never be happy with their long-term progress.

KPIs and goals

For anyone who isn't familiar: key performance indicators (KPIs) are values used to measure how well you are (or a business is) achieving objectives. Whenever you have set yourself a goal, it helps to track KPIs so you can tell if you're making good progress.

It's important to mention again that weight loss is by no means the only marker and gauge for your overall happiness and progression. Here are just a few examples of other ways you can measure your progress:

- Body fat
- Muscle mass
- Energy levels

- Overall confidence

- How your clothes feel

- Quality of sleep

- Stress levels

- Performance testing (last month I could do that; now I can do this)

There are also countless goals you can set and then track, to ensure you are on the right path. And a great way of tracking these wins or goals is ensuring you have weekly KPI targets to hit.

When you have your own business, you *need* to track KPIs – if you aren't assessing, you're guessing. If you don't use KPIs, it's likely you will go out of business or simply tread water.

Every Friday I check everything that relates to progress for our gym, including money in the bank, invoices paid, weekly direct debits, turnover for year to date, number of 28-Day Challenges sold, membership conversions, cost per lead, and any members who have left and why. Every Sunday I create new *high-value* targets for the week ahead. Every month I look at profit and loss. All this gives me a handle on the health of the business and what we most need to focus on.

Doing the same will yield similar benefits for your career. What could you track to know that you're on the right path? It might be sales calls, meetings, social media posts, tracking paid advertising, completing an assignment or project, and whether you got those big rock tasks done that day or week.

For your health and fitness journey, you can track weekly calories, steps, number of strength workouts, water intake and average hours of sleep per night (to name only a few).

When you notice that you are behind target on any of these goals, spend some extra time working at it, nail that habit down and move onto the next one. Don't overload yourself or risk increasing your stress levels – it can be detrimental to try fixing them all at once.

This is of course possible for your personal life too. For example, I became aware that I was spending too much time on my phone, especially when I was around the kids. I couldn't run the business without social media, but there is a balance to strike. I have now started limiting time on specific apps, thus reducing overall screen time for the week.

If you realise you are snacking too much, you could download an app like MyFitnessPal and track for a week or two until you get back on top of your food intake. You might identify the points in your day or week that your energy crashes, which will help you work out how to prevent that. It might have felt hard to track things like your energy and confidence levels, but you could rate these daily on a scale of one to ten. Numbers don't lie, and these numbers will help you to see what affects your energy and confidence.

This is why KPIs are so helpful – until you track and see patterns, you won't find out what you need to focus on.

Relating KPIs to goal setting is usually an easy task. Let's look at how we could relate – how much weight do you want to lose? So, how many workouts do I need to do weekly to hit my goal, how many steps per day and what is my calorie target?

How would you like to build your business, and where do you want to be in a year's time? How many weekly sales calls, social media posts, leads from ad campaigns and referrals do we need over the year to hit those targets?

It's exciting when you realise how clear you are on what you really want.

Every three months I take time out to evaluate my life and how I am spending my time, consider things I want to set in motion, plan events to look forward to as a 'reward', or simply think big. All of these help me to aim for levels I wouldn't otherwise aspire to.

It can be helpful to start with ninety-day targets – not too short, but long enough to see a real difference and embed solid habits. Once you have your ninety-day targets, you find out what you need to do to get there by working back from the end of the ninety days, breaking that time down into months, weeks and days.

Here's an example relating to our gym:

I would like thirty more monthly members in ninety days from now.

We usually lose one member a week on average – so our 'churn' rate is a healthy 2.5%. That means we need at least forty memberships sold over the next twelve weeks. I'd then look at what we need to do marketing-wise to sell forty memberships. I'd need to work out what we would need to spend to generate that outcome, and how we can make sure we take in roughly thirteen or fourteen per month, therefore three or four per week.

It's all about working *back* from the bigger goal and breaking the bigger (sometimes mentally unattainable) goals into small chunks. Otherwise, you might look ahead at your big goal and feel overwhelmed and give up.

If you want to lose a certain amount of weight or body fat, you can use a similar method. 10 kg in twelve weeks seems huge, but less than 1 kg a week will seem much more doable. It will make you more willing to do the work required.

Say you want to train for a big cycling event or marathon. Get a plan in place six to twelve months out and build up to the event. You wouldn't try to run 26 miles in the first week.

Big goals one to five years out can be motivating, but remember the factors that are likely to change your goals as you get older and your priorities change. The goals I had five years ago are very different from my current goals – I'm a different person, so I need to adapt my goals to my current situation. Maybe that 10 kg is not doable for you in 12 weeks but over 6–9 months maybe.

Maybe your lifestyle just doesn't align with the time frame.

Not willing to give up booze or nights out at weekends, it's unlikely you're going to hit those goals. I would love a shredded physique in an ideal world, but I like and value food more than I would like to be like that … so it just doesn't work.

It's vital you keep your goals realistic and achievable too. Sometimes I wonder what it would be like to grow a monster business and push to go national, with up to twenty gyms. Deep down, though, I know that I would then not spend any time at home – my relationship with Aimee would suffer and I would not see the kids grow up. I'm not willing to do that, so I'll keep my feet on the ground and create other goals to aim for.

TASK: TIME MANAGEMENT

On each social media platform you use, unfollow everyone who doesn't align with your principles and your longer-term goals.

You'll find yourself wasting less time on your phone, which will give you more time to achieve your goals.

Track the time you now spend on social media, so you can appreciate how much time you have freed up for other activities.

TASK: GET TRACKING

Write down three daily KPIs that you could track to move you forward.

Write down three to five KPIs you could assess and track weekly.

Summary

If you are one of those people who says they hate change, I want you to decide to embrace changes that benefit you, your fitness and ultimately the people around you. Remember this isn't about a complete overhaul of your life – even tiny improvements will make a big difference to your life if you maintain them over a long period. Simply force yourself to adopt new habits, and soon you will wonder how you ever managed without them.

Picturing yourself as a top athlete will help you on this journey. As soon as you start thinking you can do anything you set out to do, you will be amazed by the new goals you achieve.

Keeping everything as simple as possible underpins your success in just about anything. Stick to the basics and trust the process, and you will see better results than if you keep trying new trends.

Perhaps the most important tools to help your progress in life: setting goals and monitoring your progress. You can track just about anything, from energy levels to weight loss, from sleep quality to the success of your business. When you know exactly what you are achieving, you'll know what you need to focus on to achieve more.

SEVEN

Consistency

Doing the same stuff and sticking with what works, and doing what you need to when you said you would do it, will enable you to reach the goals you have set for yourself.

In this chapter you will find actionable strategies that will help you to maintain consistent progress. Once you get used to using these strategies, you'll find yourself thinking differently, which will make it even easier for you to make the progress you want to.

Lifestyle traffic light system

This is a system we created at DM Elite to help our members achieve consistent results. We all have different points in our life when we have varying amounts of time to focus on fitness goals. When you learn to grade your ability to commit to your goals, you will find it easier still to keep going even when you have less time, instead of giving up completely because you're not focusing 100% on your fitness.

The different levels – the ways to grade your time and commitment – are represented by the colours of traffic lights.

Red

- Damage limitation / maintenance phase
- 50% focus
- A red phase might be when you go on holiday or take time off over Christmas. Even though you're only focusing 50% on your goals, you still need to try not to undo all the good work you've already put in.

Amber

- Steady and sustainable phase
- 75% focus
- This is where you adopt the 1% better mindset and make small, marginal gains, which give you great progress in the long run. You only need to make

a small deficit in calories – one you can maintain forever, without thinking you're really giving anything up. Goals take a little longer to hit.

Green

- All-or-nothing / full-systems-go mentality
- 100% focus
- This might be in the lead-up to a time or event you particularly want to be in great shape for. You commit to a bigger calorie deficit and get faster results, but this is a tougher process that is harder to maintain longer term. Aim for 4–6 weeks at a time maximum.

As you can see, the sweet spot is amber. We would suggest there would be windows in each though. An example of a pattern for a whole year:

1. 4–8 weeks red

2. 4–8 weeks green

3. 36–44 weeks amber

I recommend this system to 90% of our members.

The red gives you the opportunity to down tools without totally stopping. For example, you may not worry too much about food or calories, but you may keep steps up and do the odd workout. You still need to keep a close eye on the longer term and the work it will require when you get back to amber/green.

At green, you achieve your best regarding calories, steps and regular training, with no junk food or booze, as you are so focused on the event you are working towards. You know this will be a bit of a battle and you cannot keep it up long term.

Personally, I stick with amber for most of the year, with maybe one or two weeks in red or green. I enjoy training for the mental health benefits, so I never want to stop that. I also do not drink, so that does a lot of the heavy lifting for me, but I enjoy giving myself a break when it comes to food.

Similar to the 'Getting 1% better' section covered earlier, amber is teaching us about delayed gratification.

One pound of weight loss per week might not feel a lot to you when starting out. If you stick at it for a year, though, you will lose 52 lb.

Similarly, if you had invested £1,000 in Apple twenty-five years ago, it would now be worth £632,000.

I hope this helps illustrate the power behind simply waiting. You can achieve bigger results by taking your time and being consistent. People often flip between red and green, repeatedly going from one extreme to another, but sticking at amber achieves long-lasting success.

Most people are impatient for results, but that also makes it harder for the mind to adjust, which can be counterproductive. An example is when lottery winners can't handle the big win and the changes in their lives, with some ending up bankrupt. Similarly, we've all seen people lose a drastic amount of weight within a short period, then soon after they revert to point A (and probably feel worse for it).

When you are willing to wait, you will keep the money in the bank or the weight off. It is not so much about the result or how to get there. It's staying there and maintaining your progress then pushing forward again.

Are you expanding or contracting?

We all make hundreds of decisions every day, but you don't need to worry about making the best choice every single time. That just will not happen and there's always a balance to strike. If you make 70% of your decisions in line with what you want over a set period, you will be on the right path. You often need that other 30% to keep an element of enjoyment and what you like. You may want to lose weight and tone up, but you also need to have a life and be able to enjoy what you enjoy. If you like having a few beers at the weekend while you watch the football or a night out with friends here and there, that's totally cool. That balance will enable you to keep going.

If you maintain a longer-term 70/30 or 80/20 balance, you will very likely be happier and better off in the longer term than a person who dips in and out of a restrictive, all-or-nothing approach to dieting and exercise. That person may drop a stone in a month, but training and eating 800–1,000 calories can be very hard to sustain.

The decisions you make every day will either be pushing you closer to your goals or driving you further away. This is known as expanding or contracting.

One thing's for sure: you would not be taking the time to read this book if you were contracting, so well done for getting to this point. Hopefully this book has made you question a few things about your life and your fitness journey, and you have expanded your mindset as a result.

CASE STUDY: LISA PENCHION

Lisa says she has never loved gyms. She had had gym memberships but could never break the cycle of signing up, going a few times then losing motivation and giving up. After a friend recommended DM Elite's 28-Day Challenge, she agreed to give it a go, although she couldn't see herself doing more than those 28 days.

Lisa admits she felt so apprehensive, she almost didn't make it to her first session. She was amazed by how welcome she felt, though, and left the gym on a high after her first session. She says the following sessions were the same – hard work but enjoyable.

Lisa joined up after the 28 days and says the gym soon became a way of life for her. She saw the gym as her new way to socialise and found herself training five or six times a week. Before long, she hardly recognised herself.

Lisa says her whole outlook on fitness has changed, to the point where she agreed to join the DM Elite team, despite not having been looking to change jobs. Now she can hardly believe how much she enjoys her work in an industry she has become passionate about. Her favourite thing about her new role is watching and helping others with their own fitness journeys.

Know your 3 Ps

You have probably heard the saying 'Fail to prepare, prepare to fail'. Plans don't always work, but *planning* does.

If you are in constant reactive mode, spinning plates while you try and keep your life on track, it's very likely you're not making any progress. Maybe you cannot get to the gym, or you struggle to make time for what you know is important. Then you need to look at slowing down a bit and planning, so that you can speed back up again.

Like most people, I have a busy life. As well as running our business, with five staff members I need to make sure we can pay every month, we have two young girls and our own family goals to hit. If I didn't plan, instead waiting for life to hit me at the start of each week, I know I'd get nowhere. If I had woken up today without a plan to write this section of the book, I know I would not have done it. There were many points in writing this book where it got tough, especially due to external pressures, and I sometimes felt like giving up. But adjusting my approach and sticking to smaller, more frequent writing sessions helped me to keep going.

Time is the one thing you can't get back, so it's critical you plan your time carefully. If you are tight for time, losing time or blaming busyness for not getting important things done, then you need to focus more on scheduling. The most successful people in any walk of life plan their schedules carefully and are super-efficient with their time. They do what they need to do and focus on high-value tasks rather than on endless to-do lists.

Think of going into every day or week having planned your 3 Ps – the personal, professional and physical areas of your life. Here are examples of all the questions I consider in each area:

Personal

- What do I want to do for myself and my family?

- How do I allocate time off and down time with the kids and their activities?

- What do I do that's fun for me so I ensure I always have stuff to look forward to?

- How do Aimee and I ensure we get a break from thinking about the business?

- How do I develop myself personally – do I read, listen to podcasts or have a coach who keeps me on track? Should I do a degree later in life?

- What steps can you put in place to make sure this stuff is looked after and you stick to your plan?

Professional

- What are my dedicated timebound tasks?

- What are the critical things I can do this week to move me closer to my bigger goal?

- How do I prepare myself to make sure I am where I need to be energy- and confidence-wise so I can fulfil my day-to-day role?

Physical

- How am I looking after my own physical health?

- Should I have a personal trainer or go to the gym?
- How do I make non-negotiable time to look after my own physical and mental health?

I want to emphasise the importance of the final point here. Your physical and mental health are your number-one asset. For most people, it's not until they face serious health issues that they appreciate the full value of good health. If you don't prioritise your own health, it won't look after itself. And if you are unhappy, struggling with poor physical and mental health due to not putting yourself first, you will no longer be able to look after everyone else.

Too often, people focus on only one of these areas. For example, you see lots of people who are in shape but have no real drive in their career. You see successful employees or entrepreneurs who put all their time into being a success but neglect how they look and feel. There are also times where I don't focus completely on my own training because I am flat out with leading the team or working on something new for the business.

It can be hard to nail all the 3 Ps at once, but that's OK. Focus on as many of the points as you can, and you will start to see your life improve. Remember that if you are at least conscious of all your personal, professional and physical priorities, in time you will be able to look after all of them. And if you observe the 3 Ps every day and every week, after a while they will look after themselves.

Once you know what you want to do on a daily and weekly basis, you only need to make sure you do it. There are always things you can do to reduce the friction that could inhibit your motivation. Here are just a few examples:

- If you plan to get up early to go to the gym or workout, get everything ready the night before. Lay all your gym stuff out, pack your bag and prep your food and drinks. When I do this, not only does it increase the chances I'll get to the gym early, but I can sleep better, not stressing when I'm half-awake in the morning about whether I'll forget something.

- If you are tracking your nutrition and aiming for a daily calorie deficit, preparing your breakfast and lunch one day ahead will make your plans much easier to achieve. If you're then running late in the morning, it's much less likely you'll be tempted to eat an unhealthy breakfast then grab a high-calorie meal deal for lunch.

- Make sure you plan ahead, allocating specific times in the week that you *know* you'll keep clear to go to the gym. If you don't, you'll keep finding yourself feeling too busy and telling yourself you'll go the next day.

- If you can't find any gaps during the week ahead, perhaps due to work meetings or childcare commitments, plan to get to the gym before the day starts on specific days of the week. This will give you more energy and drive for the rest of the day, increasing your motivation to do the same again.

- If you know you're drinking too much on weekends, book gym sessions for Saturday or Sunday morning, or both. That reduces the temptation to drink the night before, especially when you think about how great you will feel after working out instead of feeling tired and hungover.

It's fine to be spontaneous sometimes, and we need to keep enjoying life. But planning ahead and focusing on the 3 Ps will serve you well over a longer period, and there's no doubt that you will enjoy life even more once you are feeling fitter and trimmer.

Over time you will become more efficient in maintaining your 3 Ps, which will make it much easier for you to achieve your lower limit and even your upper limit, as we discussed in the first part of this book. You'll suddenly find you can easily do things that used be a challenge.

Treat your body like a bank account

The more you withdraw from your bank account, the less you have left to spend. The more deposits you make, the more you save. When you save money, it compounds over time. Similarly, when you do small bits of extra work over time, it compounds the results, and the same goes for your body and fitness.

One of my old football coaches used to run the legs off us at the end of every session. We knew it was coming and would moan before it happened, but we felt great once it was done. As our coach said, we then had 'money in the bank, ready for a rainy day', which we could use at the end of a match when the other team was tiring. We would be fitter and have a stronger mindset than all the other teams that weren't doing this. It's only really now that I fully appreciate the value of this discipline, and I now use the same mindset in everything I do.

If you double down on habits over days, weeks and months, you will experience truly life-changing results. Just make sure you keep making enough deposits – eating the right food, getting enough sleep, etc – so you don't end up broke.

You get what you focus on

We've already covered how your habits will change your results. You can't decide now on everything that will happen in your life, but you can decide on your habits, and they will dictate your future.

We've also considered the benefits of changing your mindset, and I want to take this now to another level – the benefits of being obsessed about what you really want to achieve in the longer term. Obsession and focusing on the bigger picture will help in getting you where you need to be. Obsession can be seen as a negative, but I see it as a huge positive. In fact, I believe that the most successful people are at least in part obsessed about what they want to achieve. Now it's time for you to get obsessed about yourself, your mindset, your lifestyle and your health.

If you are willing to push yourself, and you allow yourself to focus completely, to the point of obsession, you will be able to achieve goals you otherwise might not even have aimed for. Aim high, while still keeping your goals within reach – there's no point in obsessing about the unachievable.

For example, I couldn't open twenty gyms by this time next year. When I played football, I knew I wouldn't get to play for Man United. I did, though, achieve goals that I obsessed about. While I was still at school, all I thought about was becoming a professional football player and playing for Ross County. I thought about little else for five or six years. I was constantly thinking about training, the next game and what I could have done better in the previous game. I obsessed about my diet, I didn't go out drinking all the time or smoke like a lot of kids my age, and my weekends were consumed by training and matches.

It worked. I debuted at seventeen and played around fifty times for Ross County. I got there through laser focus on my end goal.

I also have to add that after I had done all I needed, I got complacent. I had the amateur mindset rather than the mindset of a top athlete, so I didn't have the direction to keep building on what I had achieved. My focus changed from expansion mode to protection mode, with me only trying to stay where I was, so I ended up contracting and going backwards.

When I was about twenty-two years old, I was now part-time with Elgin City in League 2. The previous season we just missed out for promotion through the play offs but I personally won some awards at the club as well as being nominated a second time by peers and players from other clubs into Team of the Season for the league, the first time being at Peterhead a few years before.

Coming into the new season, I was obsessed about getting in it for a third time. To make things even more exciting (well, not as a fan), Rangers were demoted to our league. Scottish internationalists and some big names were now in the league, so I challenged myself personally to have a real go at the season ahead, and hopefully make the PFA Team again as I saw Rangers being in the league as an even bigger honour.

At the end of the season, I made it in and, what is better, I was one of the four players in the league nominated for Player of the Season for the league. The season literally went exactly how I imagined personally.

Think about your own personal goal setting. What are you visioning every day? What gets you focused and out of bed every morning? What are your biggest achievements to date? You have probably had the discipline to achieve massive goals in other areas of your life. Now you need to find ways to attribute the same mindset and drive to your current lifestyle.

After my successes in football, my obsession changed to business. I started working with guys like Paul Mort as I did not want to be just another personal trainer doing only enough to get by. I wanted to be the best and build a real career in the industry.

In 2015 Paul asked me to future pace. He told me to consider what I wanted from the business – not only in relation to numbers and money, but in how I wanted to live my life. I laid out a number of clear priorities, including my wife not needing to work if she wanted to bring up our kids on our own terms, and that I wanted to build a business, employ a team and not have to rely on my football wage for income. I knew I wanted to create a community of like-minded people, and to build something unique to our local market. I knew all this was doable if I worked to my strengths and fully focused on my end goals. I knew that I had to get out of my comfort zone, and I knew I had to make sure I was never the smartest guy in the room, instead always looking up and learning from other people.

When I started out, lots of other trainers were out-performing me. They included Greg, who was in the early stages of building a gym equipment company. His company, BLK BOX, is now huge and supplies lots of gyms and premiership football teams with some of the smartest equipment on the market. I was bamboozled by Greg's numbers and goals. That made me think bigger – I knew I could achieve something similar, in my own way.

When you go to the gym, you will see people at higher levels of fitness, but don't let that be a barrier. Use it as a goal to motivate and inspire you to reach the same levels. Remember that those people would at some point have started exactly where you are now.

Think of where you're at now as a measure of what you have invested time and focus in over the past six months to a year. If you want to change your current reality, then change your current habits and give it time. You won't get anywhere if you make only short-term changes then give up if you don't achieve results.

Your results reflect how you have chosen to live over a long period of time – your priorities, your habits and who you have surrounded yourself with. To get to where you want to go, you need to focus on your long-term goals.

Your results are a direct reflection of your actions and priorities.

CASE STUDY: MARY MACFARLANE

Mary had attended various classes and gyms and been trained by different trainers before joining our gym, but she says she has never felt more connected with her fitness and wellbeing than she does now.

Mary first came to us when we were starting out. She recognises that I knew from the start the type of business I wanted to create and develop, and that I have remained focused throughout.

Starting her days with 6am sessions kickstarts each day in the most positive way possible, making her feel ready to take on whatever the day is going to bring. She maintains that feeling good in ourselves helps us with every aspect of life, and that physical, mental and financial wellbeing are all interrelated.

Mary says, 'If we can get each area to be as strong as possible then I think that can only be a good thing for living the best life we can.'

Summary

To get where we want, we need to be consistent. Keep that ball rolling and do your best not to break the chain. The most successful people develop more resilience in overcoming obstacles and reacting more effectively to challenging situations, and they simply do not stop.

It is easy to start new things, but it's harder to see them through. Sometimes life just gets in the way and you lose focus. Hopefully now, though, you have a new perspective on longer-term thinking and on the benefits of doubling down daily on your actions and habits. Whatever your goals, you *need* to go all in. Learn how to stick with repeated actions to master what you want to achieve.

Short-term thinking delivers only short-term results. We have all experienced that.

You'll achieve your biggest wins when you keep the big picture in your mind, accepting that sometimes you need to be happy with delayed gratification. The feeling of achievement when you reach your long-term goals, when you're feeling so much better than before, will make it worth every effort and every second of time you have invested.

Remember that your body is like a bank account. If you develop and maintain long-term habits, you will enjoy the compounded effects. Be obsessed and focused on what you really want, and you will achieve real, long-lasting results.

Conclusion

I hope you now have a sound understanding of my ethos and how that translates to my way of coaching. I hope you have been able to relate my own challenges to your own life, whether you have struggled with your health and fitness, or your mindset, or if you have prioritised your career or other people above your own energy, confidence and goals.

'I'll start next Monday' is not a throwaway saying. It's a limiting mindset and approach to life that I want to help you change. I want to help you develop a new mindset that propels long-lasting change in you, your health and your lifestyle. You don't need to try to action everything in this book at once. Simply having overall awareness of what you need to focus on will make a significant difference to what you can achieve.

I take pride in being different in my approach, in everything from my own fitness to helping others improve theirs, from being a parent to how I run my business. To become different, you need to think and act differently. Whether relating to your fitness, your career or your whole lifestyle, this mindset works and will help you to improve.

You may want to lose weight. Perhaps you want to transform your thinking and day-to-day actions through your fitness. Maybe you need to get fitter and drop some body fat for your long-term health, especially so you're not susceptible to health conditions as you get older. Whatever your priority, it's likely you're tired of stopping and starting, and you want to find something that works for you and makes your life better. There will be something there for you, but the key is it starts with *you*.

Whatever you want to achieve will take not only work but also a certain way of thinking and of dealing with problems and stresses. You will need to plan and always look forward, future pace, goal set and have daily tasks that move the needle ever so slightly. I of course can't guarantee that reading this book will solve problems and change your life. Use the principles you have read about and find what works for you. Then implementing the actions in this book will be vital in achieving results.

My way is certainly not the only way, but I know it works. I have practised all these methods for ten years now, using these skillsets and mindsets on my own life as well as in helping the people I have worked with since setting up my own gym.

If you need to ask for help personally or need specific personal coaching or direction, please visit our gym in Inverness, where we strive to offer the best in-person coaching available; alternatively I also offer personal coaching online for anyone looking for more accountability and direct help in any of the areas covered in this book.

To get in touch with me personally, reach out to me at dan@dmelite.co.uk.

To join our gym, visit our website: www.dmelite. co.uk.

Thanks for reading, and good luck on your journey.

Resources

Clear, J, *Atomic Habits* (Random House Business, 2018)

Jorgenson, E, *The Almanack of Naval Ravikant: A Guide to Wealth and Happiness* (Magrathea Publishing, 2020)

Mark Fisher on Instagram: @markfisherhumanbeing

Paul Mort on Instagram: @paulmort1

Acknowledgements

I would like to thank everyone who has been part of the journey to date. First Aimee for all your support, encouragement and belief to follow through on our plans and ideas since we started the business. Although I get most of the credit, without Aimee's conviction and gut instinct, DM Elite wouldn't be what it is today. Thanks also to all our staff members for giving me the time to take on this project.

A big thank-you to Mum and Dad for trusting my judgement as I grew up. Thanks to all my family for being so supportive.

A huge thank-you to all clients that have been with me or the gym over the past ten years. It has been a blast, and I appreciate everyone who has trusted me to help them on their path to a healthier life.

Thanks too to all the beta readers who helped me with the book writing process – your time and help is much appreciated, and your insight has improved the finished product.

Without all of you, this book would not have been possible.

The Author

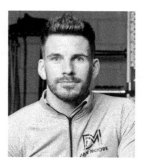 Dan is owner of Dan Moore Elite Training, Inverness, having founded the gym in 2016 and having been in the fitness industry since 2011. After being a professional football player at Ross County for five years, Dan continued to play football at a professional level part-time and stopped playing aged 30. His main drive now is helping people. Together with his wife Aimee and staff, he has helped more than 1,000 people at Dan Moore Elite Training and continues to offer the highest standard of personal training. He also coaches people online from all over the country, in personal training and lifestyle and mindset coaching, using principles he adopted in his

own life as an athlete, business owner and parent. Dan firmly believes you need to look after your health and mindset across all areas of life. His overriding ambition is to inspire people to achieve what they want to achieve and do what they have said they will do. In his spare time Dan loves spending time with his girls Beau and Macy; walking his dog, Rio; and watching his favourite football teams, Rangers and Manchester United.

To connect with Dan or contact him for more help:

- ⊕ www.dmelite.co.uk
- ▉ www.facebook.com/danielmoorept
- ◎ @imdanmoore
- ✉ dan@dmelite.co.uk